NEW DEVELOPMENTS IN MEDICAL RESEARCH

THORACIC LYMPHADENOPATHY

NEW DEVELOPMENTS IN MEDICAL RESEARCH

Additional books and e-books in this series can be found on Nova's website under the Series tab.

NEW DEVELOPMENTS IN MEDICAL RESEARCH

THORACIC LYMPHADENOPATHY

VIKAS PATHAK
EDITOR

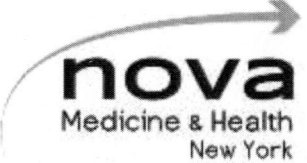

Copyright © 2020 by Nova Science Publishers, Inc.

All rights reserved. No part of this book may be reproduced, stored in a retrieval system or transmitted in any form or by any means: electronic, electrostatic, magnetic, tape, mechanical photocopying, recording or otherwise without the written permission of the Publisher.

We have partnered with Copyright Clearance Center to make it easy for you to obtain permissions to reuse content from this publication. Simply navigate to this publication's page on Nova's website and locate the "Get Permission" button below the title description. This button is linked directly to the title's permission page on copyright.com. Alternatively, you can visit copyright.com and search by title, ISBN, or ISSN.

For further questions about using the service on copyright.com, please contact:
Copyright Clearance Center
Phone: +1-(978) 750-8400   Fax: +1-(978) 750-4470   E-mail: info@copyright.com.

NOTICE TO THE READER

The Publisher has taken reasonable care in the preparation of this book, but makes no expressed or implied warranty of any kind and assumes no responsibility for any errors or omissions. No liability is assumed for incidental or consequential damages in connection with or arising out of information contained in this book. The Publisher shall not be liable for any special, consequential, or exemplary damages resulting, in whole or in part, from the readers' use of, or reliance upon, this material. Any parts of this book based on government reports are so indicated and copyright is claimed for those parts to the extent applicable to compilations of such works.

Independent verification should be sought for any data, advice or recommendations contained in this book. In addition, no responsibility is assumed by the Publisher for any injury and/or damage to persons or property arising from any methods, products, instructions, ideas or otherwise contained in this publication.

This publication is designed to provide accurate and authoritative information with regard to the subject matter covered herein. It is sold with the clear understanding that the Publisher is not engaged in rendering legal or any other professional services. If legal or any other expert assistance is required, the services of a competent person should be sought. FROM A DECLARATION OF PARTICIPANTS JOINTLY ADOPTED BY A COMMITTEE OF THE AMERICAN BAR ASSOCIATION AND A COMMITTEE OF PUBLISHERS.

Additional color graphics may be available in the e-book version of this book.

Library of Congress Cataloging-in-Publication Data

Names: Pathak, Vikas, MD, Riverside Health System, Newport News, Virginia, USA, editor. |
Title: Thoracic Lymphadenopathy
Description: New York: Nova Science Publishers, [2019] | Series: New Developments in Medical Research | Includes bibliographical references and index.
Identifiers: LCCN 2019954061 (print) | ISBN 9781536167009 (paperback) |
  ISBN 9781536167016 (adobe pdf)

Published by Nova Science Publishers, Inc. † New York

*To my parents Harekrishna and Saroj Pathak
who gave their life to work to make my life better.*

My wife Riva, who gave up her career to make my mine.

*My children Prithvi and Bhumi
who I owe uncountable weekends and holidays.*

CONTENTS

Preface		ix
Chapter 1	Anatomy of Mediastinal and Hilar Lymph Nodes *Christopher Walker and Vikas Pathak*	1
Chapter 2	Lung Cancer *Upendra R. Kaphle*	11
Chapter 3	Metastatic Cancers *Hyun S. Kim, Javeryah Safi and Danai Khemasuwan*	23
Chapter 4	Lymphoma *Santosh Nepal*	43
Chapter 5	Infectious Diseases *Fahad Gul and Abesh Niroula*	51
Chapter 6	Sarcoidosis *Christina Mutch and Vikas Pathak*	67
Chapter 7	Interstitial and Occupational Lung Diseases *Darrin Hursey, Michael Shallcross and Vikas Pathak*	77

Chapter 8	Miscellaneous Disorders Affecting Thoracic Lymph Nodes *Samer Taj-Eldin*	**91**
Chapter 9	Role of EBUS/EUS in the Diagnosis of Mediastinal and Hilar Lymphadenopathy *Raju Bishwakarma Century and Vikas Pathak*	**99**
Chapter 10	Mediastinoscopy for the Diagnosis of Mediastinal and Hilar Lymphadenopathy *Mary K. Bryant and Trevor C. Upham*	**123**
About the Editor		**141**
Index		**143**
Related Nova Science		**155**

PREFACE

Thoracic lymphadenopathy consists of mediastinal and/or hilar lymphadenopathy. Thoracic lymph nodes are anatomically one of the most complex groups of the lymphatic network in the body and describing them could be nerve wracking if there is no proper understanding of the locations, its systemic divisions and its significance in diseased states. Thoracic lymphadenopathy is one of the most common radiological findings seen on the CT scan of thorax. The incidence of these findings have particularly increased in the era of lung cancer screening with low dose CT scan of the chest. The differential diagnosis for mediastinal and hilar lymphadenopathy is broad and spans from being reactive to benign disease to lung cancer or metastatic cancer.

In this book, we have tried to simplify the lymph node stations based on the latest IASLC guidelines, done a very comprehensive review about mediastinal and hilar lymphadenopathy in different disease states and provided the pathway to diagnosis.

This book also gives a detailed account of noninvasive testing including CT chest and PET CTs. This book also discusses in detail the advanced endoscopic and non-endoscopic procedures like EBUS-TBNA, EUS and Mediastinoscopy that we have at our disposal for the diagnosis of thoracic lymphadenopathy. The indications, contraindications, sensitivity and specificity of each procedure is discussed in detail.

In: Thoracic Lymphadenopathy
Editor: Vikas Pathak

ISBN: 978-1-53616-700-9
© 2020 Nova Science Publishers, Inc.

Chapter 1

ANATOMY OF MEDIASTINAL AND HILAR LYMPH NODES

Christopher Walker[1], DO and Vikas Pathak[2], MD

[1]Campbell University School of Osteopathic Medicine, Fayetteville, North Carolina, US
[2]Riverside Regional Medical Center, Newport News, Virginia, US

INTRODUCTION TO LYMPH NODES AND LYMPHADENOPATHY

The lymph nodes are organized lymphoid structures throughout the body that filter lymphatic fluid and feature immune cells used in physiologic and pathologic responses. A simplistic description of this process may sound like this: Lymphatic fluid passes into each lymph node from afferent lymphatic vessels, and is exposed to B cells in the lymph node cortex, and to T cells deeper in the lymph node paracortex. Lymphatic fluid reaches the deepest part of the lymph node, the medulla, which is rich with lymphocytes, histiocytes, and antibody secreting plasma cells.

Fluid finally exits the lymph node through efferent vessels and proceeds to eventually reach lymphatic ducts, which drain into the venous system.

It is this process in which immune cells detect foreign proteins and signs of inflammation and generate responses [1].

Lymphadenopathy is a condition in which there is an abnormal increase in size of lymph nodes, if the size of the lymph node is ≥ 10mm as seen on the chest imaging.

Typically, lymphadenopathy is associated with the presence of pathology resulting in cellular debris, inflammation, or cellular proliferation. While the lymphatic system is diffuse and located throughout the body, it acts in a regional manner, draining local tissues. As a result, the location of lymphadenopathy is dependent on where pathology is present.

Within the thorax, lymphadenopathy is commonly associated with numerous pathologies including lung cancers, lymphoma, infections, and sarcoidosis, amongst other causes. In diagnosing and evaluating any such disorder, biopsies of the lymph nodes can have immeasurable value. Thus, it is crucial to have a firm understanding of where lymph nodes are located and how they may be reached.

There are multiple methods of identifying lymph nodes and grouping them based on anatomic location and drainage pathways. First it is important to define the regions being discussed. The mediastinum is commonly defined as the thoracic space between the pleural sacs bound anteriorly by the sternum and posteriorly by the thoracic vertebrae and extending from the thoracic inlet to the diaphragm. It is divided by a transverse plane through the manubriosternal junction and lower surface of the fourth thoracic vertebra into the superior mediastinum and inferior mediastinum.

The mediastinum merges into the interstitial pleural tissue as it extends beyond each pulmonary hilum. A 'station' is a collection of lymph nodes in a particular anatomic location.

MEDIASTINAL LYMPH NODES

The lymph nodes within the mediastinum have been mapped extensively in the past using various methodologies and grouping strategies.

In 2009, the International Association for the Study of Lung Cancer proposed an updated international lymph node map for the seventh edition of the TNM classification of lung cancer. This particular map sought to resolve discrepancies between historical maps, provide precise anatomic definitions for 14 lymph node stations, and group those stations into 7 zones for further classification.

These zones include the *supraclavicular, upper, aortopulmonary, subcarinal, lower, hilar/interlobar,* and *peripheral* zones, and were created for the purpose of prognostic analysis, rather than for nomenclature purposes [2].

Each lymph node station has defined anatomic borders that distinguish them from other stations. Some anatomic variation can be expected to exist between patients, however these recommendations apply for most patients. Stations 1, 2, and 4 are subdivided into 1R, 1L, 2R, 2L, and 4R, 4L representing stations on the right and left, respectively. Station 3 is subdivided into stations 3a and 3p representing anterior and posterior stations, respectively. The lymph node stations progress anatomically from superior to inferior.

Drainage of the lymph nodes generally runs from distal to proximal and is regional.

Lymphatic drainage of the mediastinum tends to be ipsilateral, however this has some variability.

The superior mediastinum tends to be drained via the lymph nodes of Stations 1, 2, and 4. The anterior mediastinum drains via the lymph nodes of Stations 5 and 6. The posteroinferior mediastinum is drained via the lymph nodes of Stations 7, 8, and 9 [3]. Understanding the locations of these Stations and the regions with which they are associated is crucial to understanding how best to sample these nodes and their clinical significance.

ANATOMIC DEFINITIONS OF THE 2009 IASLC LYMPH NODE STATIONS

Station 1R and Station 1L: Low Cervical, Supraclavicular, and Sternal Notch Lymph Nodes

Station 1 lymph nodes of the supraclavicular zone are divided into 1R and 1L stations reflective of one another with the midline of the trachea serving as the midline. Station 1R and Station 1L lymph nodes are bordered by the lower margin of the cricoid cartilage superiorly, the bilateral clavicles inferiorly, and the upper border of the manubrium medially.

Station 2R and Station 2L: Upper Paratracheal Lymph Nodes

Station 2 lymph nodes of the upper zone are a collection of superior mediastinal nodes divided into stations 2R and 2L, with the left lateral border of the trachea as the separating boundary. Stations 2R and 2L are bordered superiorly by the right and left lung apices and pleura, respectively, and the upper border of the manubrium in the midline. Station 2R is bordered inferiorly by the intersection of the caudal margin of the innominate vein with the trachea. Station 2L is bordered inferiorly by the superior border of the aortic arch.

Station 3A: Prevascular Nodes and Station 3P: Retrotracheal Lymph Nodes

Station 3A and 3P lymph nodes of the upper zone are a collection of the superior mediastinum are bordered superiorly by the apex of the chest and bordered inferiorly by the carina. Station 3A is bordered anteriorly by the posterior aspect of the sternum. The posterior border of Station 3A is comprised of the anterior border of the superior vena cava on the right and the left carotid artery on the left. Station 3P lymph nodes are those located in the retrotracheal region, or the area posterior to the trachea.

Station 4R and Station 4L: Lower Paratracheal Lymph Nodes

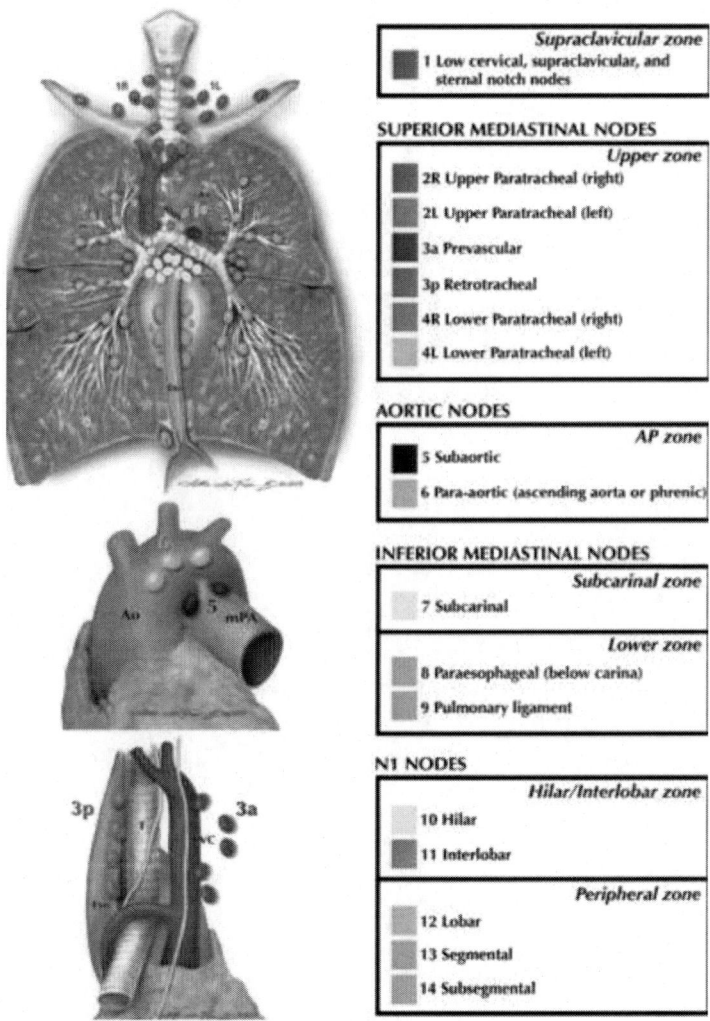

Figure 1. The International Association for the Study of Lung Cancer (IASLC) lymph node map, including the proposed grouping of lymph node stations into "zones" for the purposes of prognostic analyses (Image re-produced with permission from IASLC).

The lower paratracheal lymph nodes, known as Stations 4R and 4L are the last group of lymph nodes in the upper zone and are inferior to Station 2 lymph nodes. The left lateral wall of the trachea serves as the boundary between Stations 4R and 4L.

Station 4R is bordered by the intersection of the caudal margin of the innominate vein with the trachea superiorly, and the lower border of the azygos vein inferiorly. Station 4L is bordered by the upper margin of the aortic arch superiorly. The inferior border of Station 4L is the upper rim of the left main pulmonary artery. Station 4L extends leftward and is bordered laterally by the ligament arteriosum.

Station 5: Subaortic Lymph Nodes

Station 5 lymph nodes are located in the AP Zone, lateral to the ligament arteriosum. They are bordered superiorly by the lower border of the aortic arch, and inferiorly by the upper rim of the left main pulmonary border.

Station 6: Paraaortic Lymph Nodes

Station 6 lymph nodes are the paraaortic lymph nodes, which are also located in the AP zone. A transverse plane drawn across the upper border of the aortic arch forms the superior border. The lower border of the aortic arch forms the inferior border of the station. This station is located anteriorly and laterally to the aortic arch.

Station 7: Subcarinal Lymph Nodes

The subcarinal zone consists of the Station 7 subcarinal lymph nodes, which are a group of inferior mediastinal nodes. As its name implies, the upper border of this station is the carina. Inferiorly, Station 7 is bordered by the upper edge of the left lower lobe bronchus and the upper edge of the right bronchus intermedius, on the left and right respectively.

Station 8: Paraesophageal Lymph Nodes

Station 8 lymph nodes are inferior mediastinal node and are the first of two stations located in the lower zone. The paraesophageal lymph nodes are directly inferior to Station 7 lymph nodes and consist of the nodes adjacent to the esophagus which are not included in Station 7. Station 8 shares its upper borders with the subcarinal lymph nodes and is defined by the upper edge of the left lower lobe bronchus on the left, and the upper edge of the right bronchus intermedius on the right. The inferior border of Station 8 lymph nodes is the diaphragm.

Station 9: Pulmonary Ligament Lymph Nodes

The lower zone also includes the pulmonary ligament lymph nodes, known as Station 9. These are also inferior mediastinal nodes and lie within the pulmonary ligament. The superior border is defined by the inferior pulmonary veins, while the diaphragm delineates the inferior border of Station 9.

Station 10: Hilar Lymph Nodes

The hilar lymph nodes of Station 10 are within the hilar/interlobar zone and are adjacent to the mainstem bronchi and hilar vessels, the proximal pulmonary veins, and the main pulmonary arteries. The lower rim of the azygous vein makes the superior border of Station 10 on the right, while the upper rim of the left pulmonary artery makes the superior border of Station 10 on the left. Bilaterally, Station 10 is bordered inferiorly by the interlobar regions.

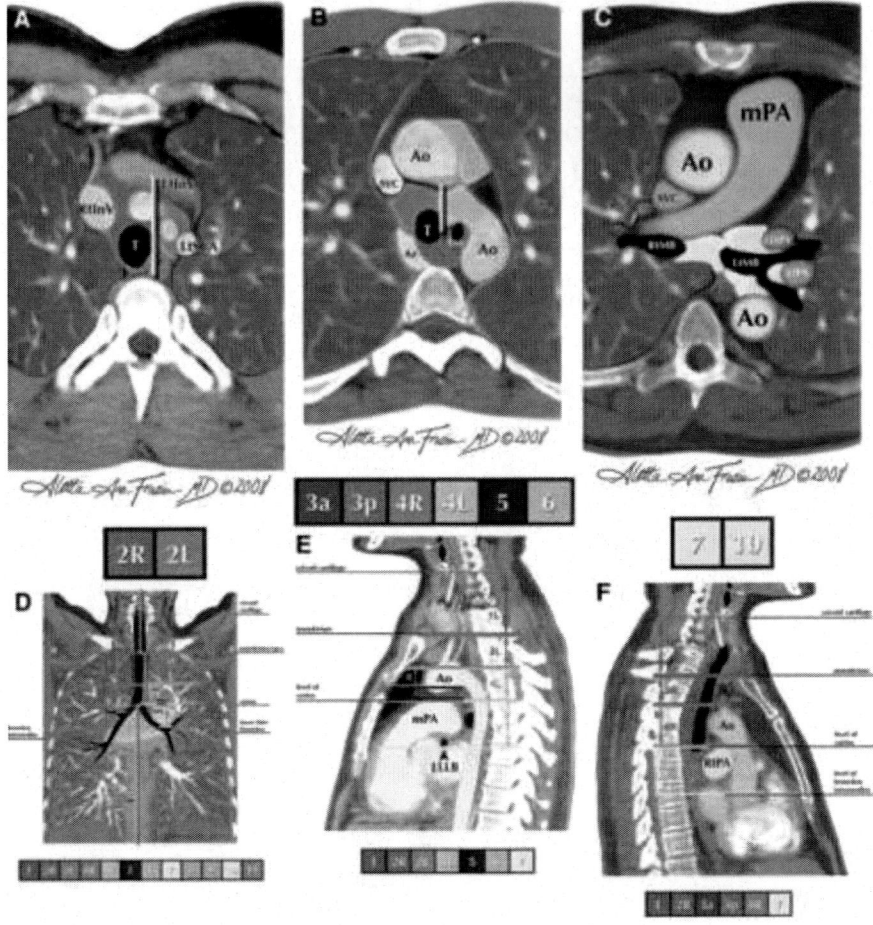

Figure 2. The International Association for the Study of Lung Cancer (IASLC) lymph node map, including the proposed grouping of lymph node stations into "zones" for the purposes of prognostic analyses (Image re-produced with permission from IASLC).

Station 11: Interlobar Lymph Nodes

The interlobar lymph nodes of Station 11 are also within the hilar/interlobar zone. These nodes are distal to the mainstem bronchi bifurcations and reside between the origins of lobar bronchi.

Station 12: Lobar Lymph Nodes

Within the peripheral zone, the lobar lymph nodes of Station 12 are the first group. Bilaterally, Station 12 lymph nodes are located adjacent to the lobar bronchi and laterality is distinguished as 12R or 12L being on the right or left, respectively.

Station 13: Segmental Lymph Nodes

Progressing through the peripheral zone, Station 13 consists of segmental lymph nodes. Station 13 is comprised of the lymph nodes lying adjacent to the segmental bronchi bilaterally. Laterality is distinguished as Station 13R on the right, or Station 13L on the left.

Station 14: Subsegmental Lymph Nodes

The final nodes of the peripheral zone are the subsegmental lymph nodes of Station 14. The lymph nodes of Station 14 are those adjacent to the subsegmental bronchi. Laterality is distinguished as Station 14R on the right, and Station 14L on the left.

REFERENCES

[1] Willard-Mack, C. L. Normal Structure, Function, and Histology of Lymph Nodes. *Toxicol. Pathol.*, 2006; 34:409 - 424.

[2] Rusch, V. W., Asamura, H., Watanabe, H., Giroux, D. J., Rami-Porta, R., Goldstraw, P. The IASLC Lung Cancer Staging Project: A Proposal for a New International Lymph Node Map in the Forthcoming Seventh Edition of the TNM Classification for Lung Cancer. *J. Thorac Oncol.*, 2009; 4(5):568 - 577.

[3] Losano Brotons, M., Bolca, C., Fréchette, É., Deslauriers, J. Anatomy and Physiology of the Thoracic Lymphatic System. *Thorac Surg. Clin. NA.*, 2012; 22: 139 - 153.

In: Thoracic Lymphadenopathy
Editor: Vikas Pathak

ISBN: 978-1-53616-700-9
© 2020 Nova Science Publishers, Inc.

Chapter 2

LUNG CANCER

Upendra R. Kaphle, MD, FCCP
Tulane University School of Medicine,
New Orleans, Louisiana, US

INTRODUCTION

The lungs have very rich lymphatic supply. The role of lymphatic system is to clear interstitial fluid from the lungs and to remove foreign particles. This pathway is also responsible for the spread of tumor from the lungs. The lymphatic system consists of parenchymal and pleural network. The pleural lymphatics course over the visceral and parietal pleural surfaces and drain into the medial aspect of the lung near the hilum, where they anastomose with the parenchymal lymphatics [1]. The parenchymal lymphatics are located in the interlobular septa and bronchovascular bundles. Multiple lymphatic channels anastomose with each other and drain sequentially into the intralobular, interlobular, lobar, and finally to the hilar nodes. This lymphatic pathway is responsible for the spread of tumor from the lung to the hilum and subsequently into the mediastinum. Hence, accurate assessment of the presence and absence of tumor in the regional lymph nodes is critical in the management of primary lung carcinoma. Though mediastinal and hilar lymphadenopathy is a very common finding in primary lung carcinoma, clinical symptoms related to lymphadenopathy is extremely uncommon. Major symptoms of lung carcinoma are related to local effects, regional or distant spread and sometimes paraneoplastic syndromes. Most of the patients with lung cancer especially small cell lung cancer have advanced disease at clinical presentation. Most common symptoms of lung cancer are cough, dyspnea, chest pain and hemoptysis (Figure 1). Since, the National Lung Screening Trial (NLST) [2] showed a 20.0% decrease in mortality from lung cancer in the low-dose CT group as compared with the radiography group in patients with high risk for lung cancer, lung cancer screening has been the standard of care. Hence, many of the asymptomatic patients are found to have abnormal imaging through annual lung cancer screening (Figure 2) or incidental detection (Figure 3) or gradually enlarging lung nodule (Figure 4) which are eventually diagnosed to have lung carcinoma.

Accurate staging of mediastinal and hilar lymph nodes plays a crucial role in identifying the best treatment plans and predicting the patient outcome. Currently used lymph node maps have been reconciled to the internationally accepted International Association for the Study of Lung Cancer (IASLC) [3] map which is based on retrospective survival analyses of international databases.

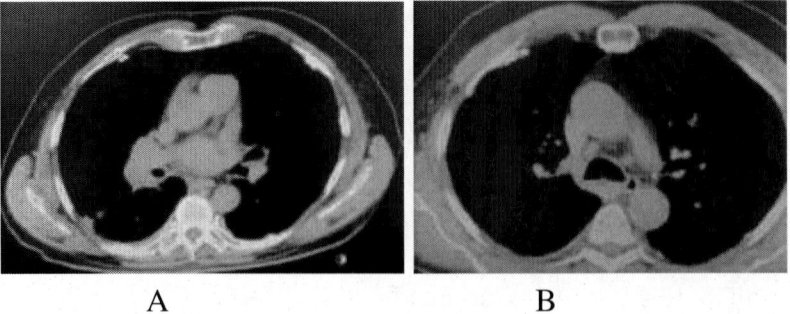

Figure 1. A 68-year-old man presented with symptoms of cough, dyspnea and hemoptysis. CT chest obtained showed 2.9 cm right hilar mass (A) with Station 4R and left lower paratracheal (4L) lymph node enlargement (B).

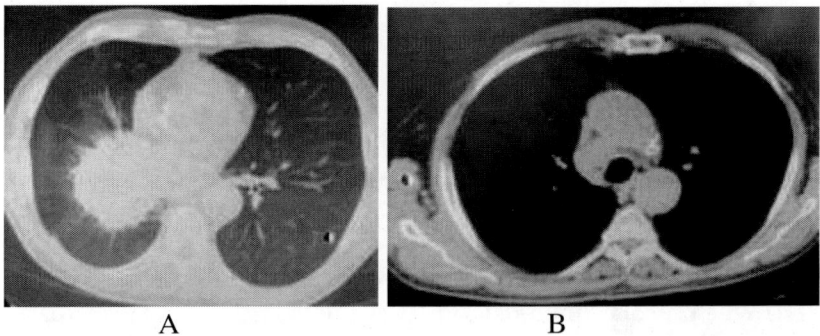

Figure 2. A 70-year-old asymptomatic 50 pack year active smoker man found to have 8 cm right lung mass (A) along with 2.2 cm right lower paratracheal (station 4R) lymph node (B) during annual lung cancer screening CT chest.

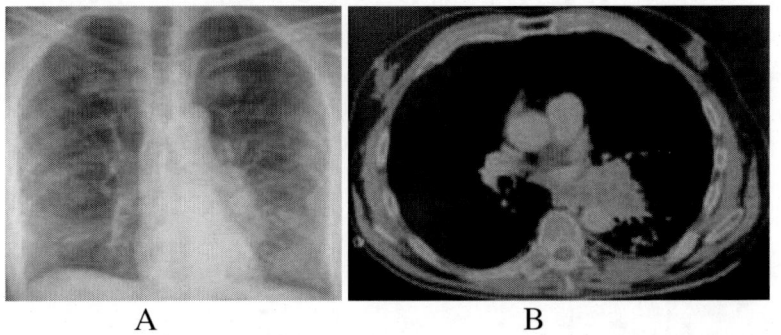

Figure 3. A 66-year-old with history of 40 pack year active smoking presented with chest wall pain. Chest X-ray (A) showed incidental left hilar mass. CT chest (B) showed 3.5 cm lung mass with mediastinal infiltration.

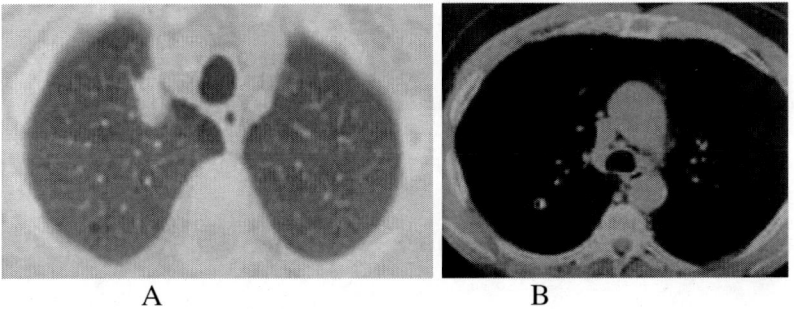

Figure 4. A 59-year-old man with gradually enlarging 2.2 cm right upper lobe lung nodule (A) along with mediastinal lymphadenopathy station 4L and 4R (B).

This internationally agreed uniform classification system is crucial for treatment planning, assessing treatment outcomes, and conducting future prospective database centered survival analyses. In the IASLC map, the 14 stations are reorganized into seven zones which extend from the supraclavicular region to the diaphragm. These lymph nodes are located in intrathoracic (mediastinal, hilar, lobar, interlobar, segmental, and subsegmental), scalene, and supraclavicular areas (Figure 5). Usually the location of the primary tumor determines the nodal pathways for mediastinal lymph node involvement [4]. Tumor in right upper lobe predominantly involves lower station 4R followed by station 2R and station 3 nodes. RUL less commonly involves stations 7, 8, and 9 nodes. Right middle lobe primary tumors most commonly involve station 7 nodes followed by station 3 and then stations (4R and 2R) nodes. Left lower lobe primary tumors most commonly involves station 7 nodes followed by near equal involvement of stations (2R, 4R, 8, 9) nodes and then involvement of station 3 nodes.

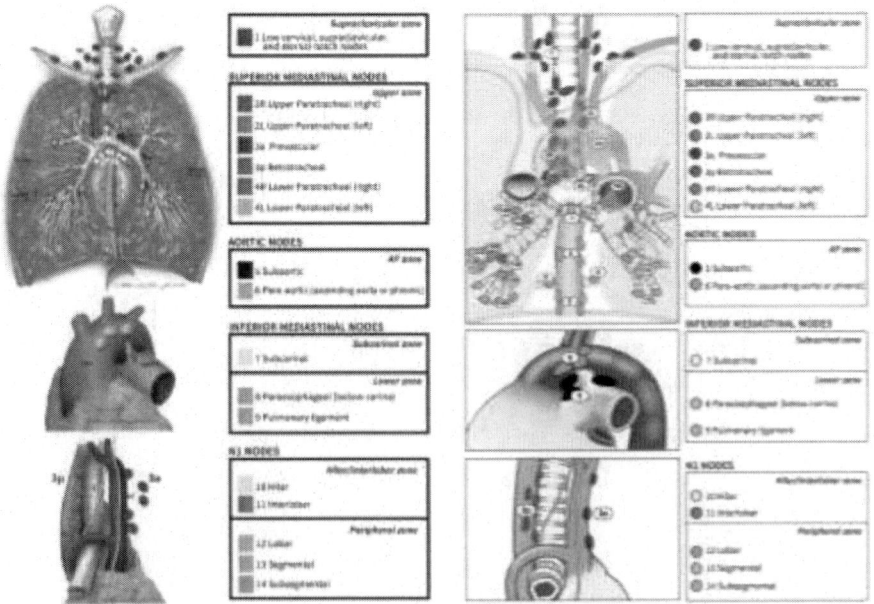

Figure 5. The International Association for the Study of Lung Cancer nodal chart with stations and zones (Image reproduced with permission from IASLC).

Tumors in left upper lobe predominantly involves the station 5 and station 6 nodes followed by station 4L. Similar to right upper lobe, left upper lobe also less commonly involves stations 7, 8 and 9 nodal stations. The left lower lobe tumors predominantly involve station 7 nodes followed by stations 4L, 5, 8, 9 nodes. Therefore, it is essential to identify the relevant lymph node regions and their relations to the primary tumor [4].

Sometimes, intrapulmonary, interlobar, and hilar lymph nodes can be bypassed to cause skip metastasis to mediastinal lymph nodes through direct lymphatic drainage. This is most commonly seen in the upper lobes tumor [5]. Rarely, a direct connection may exist between the pulmonary segments and the thoracic duct, enabling direct passage of tumor into the systemic circulation without mediastinal metastasis. Hence, once the mediastinal lymph nodes are involved, each zone can be involved and should not be neglected. Hence, systematic lymph nodes sampling should be performed for proper staging.

The Tumor, Node, Metastasis (TNM) staging system for lung cancer (NSCLC) is an internationally accepted system used to characterize the extent of disease. The current edition of the TNM staging system, effective as of January 1, 2018, categorizes tumors on the basis of primary tumor characteristics (T), the presence or absence of regional lymph node involvement (N), and the presence or absence of distant metastases (M) [6]. The overall stage of the tumor (stage I through IV) is determined by the combination of T, N, and M descriptors [6]. The classification applies to carcinomas of the lung including non-small cell carcinomas, small cell carcinomas, and bronchopulmonary carcinoid tumors. It does not apply to sarcomas and other rare tumors. It applies during clinical-diagnostic stage, surgical-pathologic stage, retreatment stage, and autopsy stage.

In this IASLC nodal nomenclature, contralateral lymph node involvement (related to primary tumor) would be classified as N3 disease (TNM classification). Involvement of mediastinal nodes, if limited to the midline stations or ipsilateral stations 2-9, would be classified as N2 disease. Involvement of station 10-14 if ipsilateral would be classified as N1 disease. Contralateral involvement of station 2, 4, 5, 6, 8, 9, 10-14 would be classified as N3. Direct extension of the primary tumor into lymph nodes is classified as lymph node metastasis.

Radiographic staging of lung cancer is performed using CT chest (including liver and adrenals), whole-body PET or integrated PET/CT which provide an assessment of tumor size (T), mediastinal node enlargement (N), and potential metastases (M) [7]. Preferably, CT chest should be obtained using intravenous contrast enhancement as it is helpful in distinguishing metastatic lymph nodes from vascular structures. There is no clear-cut size threshold for metastatic lymphadenopathy but lymph nodes of size > 1cm on short-axis diameter on transverse CT scan and the lymph nodes with fluorodeoxyglucose (FDG) uptake greater than that of mediastinal blood pool on PET imaging are considered abnormal. But, even the small or not highly FDG avid lymph nodes can be malignant. The sensitivity and specificity of CT chest and PET for identifying abnormal lymphadenopathy are (55 and 81%) and (80 and 88%) respectively. Hence, radiological staging can miss occult cancer (false negatives) and can deny potentially curative treatment (false positives). Hence, confirmation by tissue biopsy must be pursued. But, the radiological staging has its value in guiding the clinician in choosing the most optimal site for tissue sampling which should be the least invasive biopsy site with the yield of the highest possible stage.

Endobronchial ultrasound (EBUS)-directed needle aspiration has been regarded as the most commonly used minimally invasive modality with high diagnostic accuracy for systematic lymph node sampling for diagnosis and staging. Combining EBUS and Endoscopy ultrasound (EUS) results in an increased sensitivity for detecting lymph node metastases compared with EBUS alone. More invasive modalities like video-assisted thoracic surgery (VATS) and mediastinoscopy are reserved if the endosonographic approach is non-diagnostic or inaccessible for tissue sampling [8].

Distinction of lung cancer as either small cell lung cancer (SCLC) or non-small cell lung cancer (NSCLC) has a very important role for proper staging, treatment, and prognosis [9]. Approximately 95% of all lung cancers are classified as either non-small cell lung cancer (NSCLC) or small cell lung cancer (SCLC). The most common histologic categories in NSCLC are adenocarcinoma approximately 50% and squamous cell carcinomas approximately 25%. SCLC accounts for approximately 15 percent of all bronchogenic carcinoma. Other cell types comprise approximately 5 percent of malignancies arising in the lung.

Immunohistochemical (IHC) stains are used to distinguish between various types of NSCLC. Adenocarcinoma is typically positive for thyroid transcription factor (TTF-1), mucin and Napsin-A (Figure 6). Squamous cell carcinoma is typically positive for p63, p40, cytokeratin (CK) 5, 6, and CK7 (Figure 7). Adenosquamous or large cell carcinoma may have a combination of IHC staining patterns of both adenocarcinoma and squamous cell carcinoma. A limited stain of one lung adenocarcinoma marker (TTF1, Napsin A) and one squamous cell carcinoma marker (p63, p40) should suffix for differentiating most of NSCLC [10]. Small cell is usually positive for TTF1 with variable expression of other neuroendocrine markers like chromogranin, synaptophysin and CD56. But, morphology is more important than immunotype in the diagnosis of small cell carcinoma (Figure 8, 9). For patients with newly diagnosed lung carcinoma, a multidisciplinary approach that includes input from medical oncology, radiation oncology, thoracic surgery, pathology, radiology and pulmonology is recommended for formulating treatment plans.

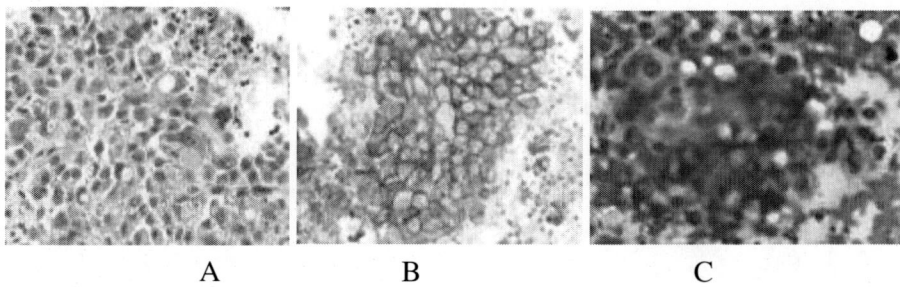

Figure 6. EBUS with transbronchial needle aspiration on Station 4L suggestive of Non-small cell lung carcinoma (NSCLC) on Cell block, H&E (A) and Cytology smear, Diff-Quick stain (C). Immunohistochemistry was positive for EP-CAM (C) favoring diagnosis of adenocarcinoma. Pictures obtained 200X magnification: (Slide courtesy: Dr. Bernardo Ruiz).

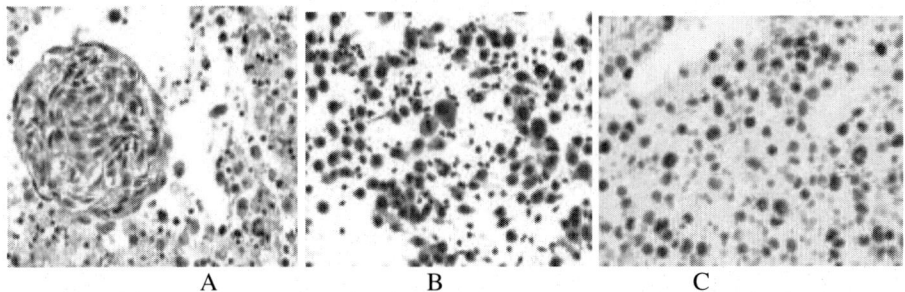

Figure 7. EBUS with transbronchial needle aspiration on Station 4R suggestive of Non-small cell lung carcinoma (NSCLC) on Cell block, H&E (A) and Cytology smear, Papanicolaou stain (B). Immunohistochemistry was positive for p63 (C) favoring diagnosis of squamous cell carcinoma. Pictures obtained 200X magnification: (Slide courtesy: Dr. Bernardo Ruiz).

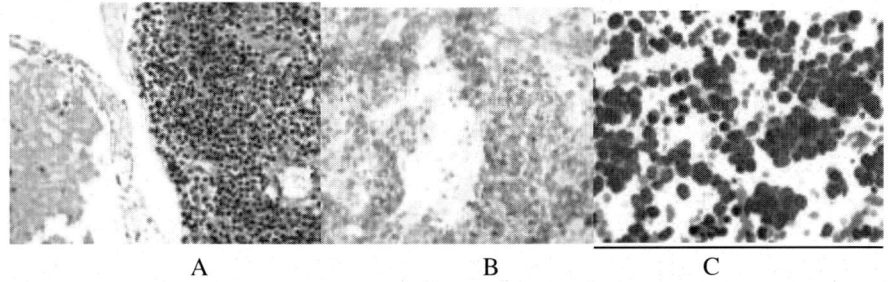

Figure 8. EBUS with transbronchial needle aspiration on station 4R suggestive of small cell carcinoma on Cell block, H&E (A) and Cytology smear, Diff-Quick stain (C). Immunohistochemistry was positive for synaptophysin (B). Pictures obtained 200X magnification: (Slide courtesy: Dr. Bernardo Ruiz).

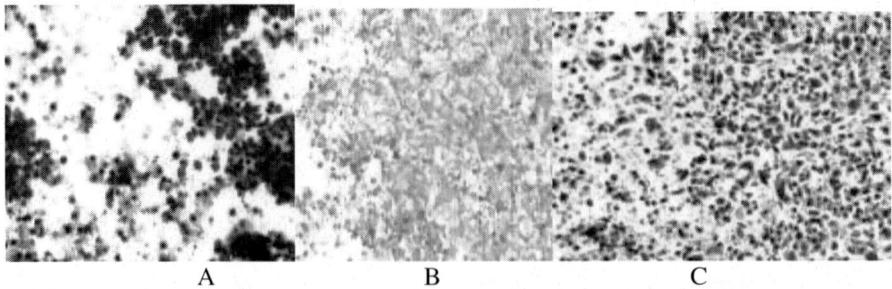

Figure 9. EBUS with transbronchial needle aspiration on Station 4L suggestive of small cell carcinoma on Cell block, H&E (A) and Cytology smear, Diff-Quick stain (C). Immunohistochemistry was positive for synaptophysin (B). Pictures obtained 200X magnification: (Slide courtesy: Dr. Bernardo Ruiz).

Patients with stage I or II NSCLC are usually treated with complete surgical resection whenever possible. Definite radiation therapy techniques with Stereotactic ablative radiotherapy (SABR), also known as stereotactic body radiation therapy (SBRT) is recommended for patients who are medically inoperable or who refuse surgery.

During surgical resection, N1 and N2 node resection and mapping should be done with a minimum of three N2 stations sampled or complete lymph node dissection. Quantifying nodal disease has prognostic impact and assists physicians in planning therapy and follow-up. Complete resection requires free margin, systematic node dissection, and the highest mediastinal node negative for tumor. If occult-positive N2 nodes is discovered at the time of surgery, planned resection should continue along with formal mediastinal lymph node dissection. If N2 disease is noted during VATS, the procedure can be stopped for induction therapy or continued depending on multidisciplinary recommendations and discussion with patient family. Postoperative adjuvant chemotherapy improves survival in patients with pathologic stage II disease.

For pathologically proven stage III NSCLC, a combined modality approach using concurrent chemoradiotherapy is generally preferred. The role of surgery in patients with pathologically documented N2 disease remains controversial. There are some suggestions regarding the role of surgery in a certain subset of patient with single-station N2 disease less than 3 cm prior to induction therapy which can be resected via lobectomy or clearance of mediastinal lymph nodes after induction chemotherapy or chemoradiation [7].

The molecular characterization of tumor tissue in patients with advanced NSCLC serves as a guidance in choosing between standard chemotherapy versus up-front targeted therapies. Specific targeted therapies have been standard therapy in patients with driver mutations like epidermal growth factor receptor (EGFR), anaplastic lymphoma kinase (ALK), ROS1, BRAF, etc. For those without driver mutations, immunotherapy such as inhibitors of programmed death 1 (PD-1) and its ligand PD-L1 are available options in certain subsets of patients [11]. Overall quality of life and progression-free survival (PFS) have improved for patients with advanced NSCLC who have specific predictive biomarkers and receive targeted therapy or immunotherapy compared with those receiving chemotherapy.

Stage IV NSCLC are generally treated with systemic therapy or a symptom-based palliative approach. Systemic chemotherapy is the mainstay component of treatment for SCLC. Thoracic radiation therapy is used in combination with chemotherapy for limited-stage disease. Prophylactic cranial irradiation decreases the incidence of brain metastases.

In conclusion, lung cancer is the leading cause of cancer deaths worldwide in both men and women [12]. The lymphatic pathway is responsible for the spread of tumor from the lung to the regional lymph nodes. Hence, systematic and complete assessment of mediastinal and hilar nodal stations is essential for accurate staging in formulating the most appropriate treatment plan and determining the prognosis.

REFERENCES

[1] Schraufnagel, D. E. Lung lymphatic anatomy and correlates. *Pathophysiology,* 2010 Sep; 17(4):337 - 43.

[2] Aberle, D. R., Adams, A. M., Berg, C. D., Black, W. C., Clapp, J. D., Fagerstrom, R. M., Gareen, I. F., Gatsonis, C., Marcus, P. M., Sicks, J. D. Reduced lung-cancer mortality with low-dose computed tomographic screening. *N Engl. J. Med.,* 2011 Aug 4; 365(5):395 - 409.

[3] Rusch, V. W., Asamura, H., Watanabe, H., Giroux, D. J., Rami-Porta, R., Goldstraw, P. The IASLC lung cancer staging project: a proposal for a new international lymph node map in the forthcoming seventh edition of the TNM classification for lung cancer. *J. Thorac Oncol.,* 2009 May; 4(5):568 - 77.

[4] Liang, R. B., Yang, J., Zeng, T. S., Long, H., Fu, J. H., Zhang, L. J., Lin, P., Wang, X., Rong, T. H., Hou, X., Yang, H. X. Incidence and Distribution of Lobe-Specific Mediastinal Lymph Node Metastasis in Non-small Cell Lung Cancer: Data from 4511 Resected Cases. *Ann. Surg. Oncol.,* 2018 Oct.; 25(11):3300 - 3307.

[5] Galbis-Caravajal, J. M., Lafuente-Sanchis, A., Estors-Guerrero, M., Martinez-Hernández, N., Fuster-Diana, C., Cremades, A., Zúñiga, Á. Topography of the sentinel node according to the affected lobe in lung cancer. *Clin. Transl. Oncol.,* 2017 Jul.; 19(7):858 - 864.

[6] Detterbeck, F. C., Boffa, D. J., Kim, A. W., Tanoue, L. T. The Eighth Edition Lung Cancer Stage Classification. *Chest,* 2017 Jan.; 151(1):193 - 203.

[7] Silvestri, G. A., Gonzalez, A. V., Jantz, M. A., Margolis, M. L., Gould, M. K., Tanoue, L. T., Harris, L. J., Detterbeck, F. C. Methods for staging non-small cell lung cancer: Diagnosis and management of lung cancer, 3rd ed: American College of Chest Physicians evidence-based clinical practice guidelines. *Chest,* 2013 May; 143(5 Suppl.):e211S-e250S.

[8] Gomez, M., Silvestri, G. A. Endobronchial ultrasound for the diagnosis and staging of lung cancer. *Proc. Am. Thorac Soc.,* 2009 Apr. 15; 6(2):180 - 6.

[9] Travis, W. D., Brambilla, E., Burke, A. P., Marx, A., Nicholson, A. G. Introduction to The 2015 World Health Organization Classification of Tumors of the Lung, Pleura, Thymus, and Heart. *J. Thorac Oncol.,* 2015 Sep.; 10(9):1240 - 1242.

[10] National Comprehensive Cancer Network (NCCN) *Clinical Practice Guidelines in Oncology, Non-Small Cell Lung Cancer,* Version 3. 2018-February 21, 2018.

[11] Gandhi, L., Rodríguez-Abreu, D., Gadgeel, S., Esteban, E., Felip, E., De Angelis, F., Domine, M., Clingan, P., Hochmair, M. J., Powell, S. F., Cheng, S. Y., Bischoff, H. G., Peled, N., Grossi, F., Jennens, R. R., Reck, M., Hui, R., Garon, E. B., Boyer, M., Rubio-Viqueira, B., Novello, S., Kurata, T., Gray, J. E., Vida, J., Wei, Z., Yang, J., Raftopoulos, H., Pietanza, M. C., Garassino, M. C. Pembrolizumab plus Chemotherapy in Metastatic Non-Small-Cell Lung Cancer. *N Engl. J. Med.,* 2018 May 31; 378(22):2078 - 2092.

[12] Torre, L. A., Bray, F., Siegel, R. L., Ferlay, J., Lortet-Tieulent, J., Jemal, A. Global cancer statistics, 2012. *CA Cancer J. Clin.,* 2015 Mar.; 65(2):87 - 108.

Chapter 3

METASTATIC CANCERS

Hyun S. Kim, MD, Javeryah Safi, MD and Danai Khemasuwan, MD
St. Elizabeth's Medical Center,
Tufts University School of Medicine, Boston, MA, US

INTRODUCTION

Mediastinal lymphadenopathy is relatively an uncommon finding in patients with extrathoracic malignancies (Figure 1). But it poses significant diagnostic dilemma for radiologists, pulmonologists, thoracic surgeons, and oncologists. The prevalence of enlarged mediastinal and hilar lymph nodes in setting of extrathoracic cancer is estimated to be approximately 2.3% [1]. This value likely underestimates the true incidence as the study utilized chest radiographs instead of more sensitive imaging modalities such as computed tomography (CT) or endobronchial ultrasound (EBUS). Enlarged mediastinal lymph nodes are often discovered as part of a staging work up at the time of diagnosis of extrathoracic malignancies and can considerably alter the staging, prognosis, and treatment strategies. Alternatively, mediastinal lymphadenopathy may be discovered by surveillance CT scans and require pathological evaluation to exclude or confirm the cancer recurrence. Other possibilities including granulomatous inflammation, indolent infections, and reactive lymphadenopathy should be included when forming differential diagnosis for mediastinal lymphadenopathy in patients with extrathoracic malignancies.

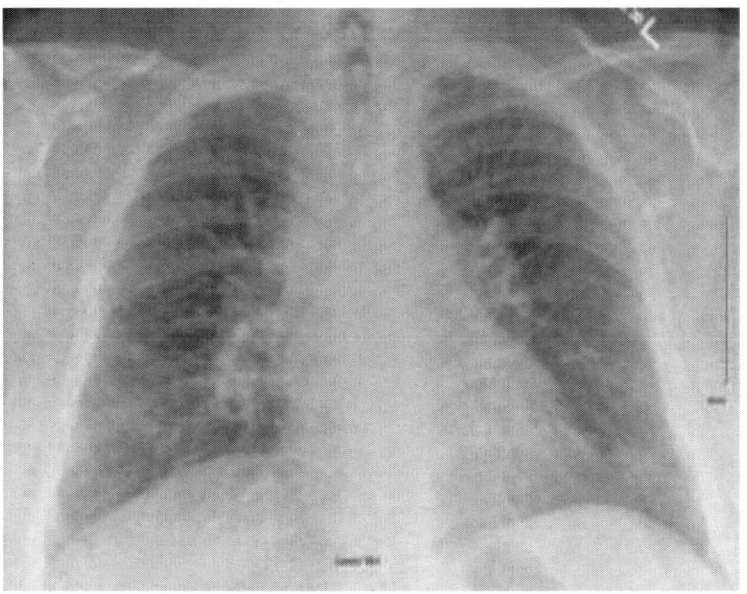

Figure 1. Posteroanterior chest radiograph of a patient with mediastinal and hilar lymphadenopathy.

ANATOMY OF MEDIASTINUM

The mediastinum is an anatomic region located between the lungs, and houses different key anatomic structures including the heart, great vessels, trachea, esophagus, thymus, thoracic duct, phrenic nerves, and the vagus nerve. It also serves as a central hub for lymphatic drainage, making mediastinum an area of concern in the setting of known malignancy. It is bordered superiorly by the superior thoracic aperture, inferiorly by the diaphragm, anteriorly by the sternum and costal cartilages, and posteriorly by the vertebrae.

The mediastinum is classically divided into three functional compartments: anterior (pre-vascular), middle (visceral), and posterior (paravertebral) mediastinum. These compartments are used to describe the location of mediastinal lesions and to facilitate the generation of differential diagnosis. The anterior mediastinum is bordered anteriorly by the sternum and costal cartilages, and posteriorly by the anterior pericardiac sac. It consists of loose connective tissue, fat, a few lymph nodes, and branches of the internal thoracic vessels. Occasionally, it can also contain the thymus gland. Several neoplastic processes can originate or invade into the anterior mediastinum. These include thymomas, lymphomas, teratomas, and other germ cell tumors. The middle mediastinum is located between the anterior and posterior mediastinum. It houses the heart and pericardium, great vessels, trachea and proximal airways, phrenic nerves, and lymphatics. Lesions found in the middle mediastinum are largely bronchogenic or pericardial cysts, but can also be from pulmonary malignancies, sarcoidosis, lymphomas, and other extrathoracic malignancies. Most of mediastinal lymph nodes reside in the anterior and middle mediastinum, thus careful attention should be given while studying computed tomography (CT) scans of patients with concerns of mediastinal malignancy. Lastly, the posterior mediastinum is bordered anteriorly by the posterior aspect of the heart and posteriorly by the vertebral bodies. It houses esophagus, descending thoracic aorta, azygous system of veins, autonomic nerves, sympathetic trunk, and lymph nodes. Lesions in the posterior mediastinum are usually neurogenic tumors or sites of extramedullary hematopoiesis. It is often very helpful to consider the location of the mediastinal lesion with symptoms, epidemiology, and demographics to generate the most likely differential diagnosis, which encompass a wide breadth of infections, inflammatory processes, and malignancies.

Due to the complexity of the lymph node anatomy in the mediastinum and the hilum, there have been many efforts to map and classify intrathoracic lymph nodes. To reconcile the differences between the two pervasive lymph node mapping m1ethods, the Naruke of the Japan Lung Cancer Society and the Mountain-Dresler modification of the American Thoracic Society, the International Association for the Study of Lung Cancer (IASLC) defined the intrathoracic lymph nodes into 14 stations according to their relationship to landmarks encountered during mediastinoscopy and thoracotomy (Figure 2) [2,3]. These stations can be further grouped into 7 zones: supraclavicular, superior mediastinal, aortopulmonary, subcarinal, inferior mediastinal, hilar, and peripheral zones [4]. This mapping method is well-incorporated into the TNM staging of non-small cell lung cancers by the American Joint Commission on Cancer (AJCC) and achieved much needed uniformity. However, IASLC lymph node mapping has not been utilized for metastatic malignancies from extrathoracic origin as its staging does not rely on any particular distribution of lymphadenopathy.

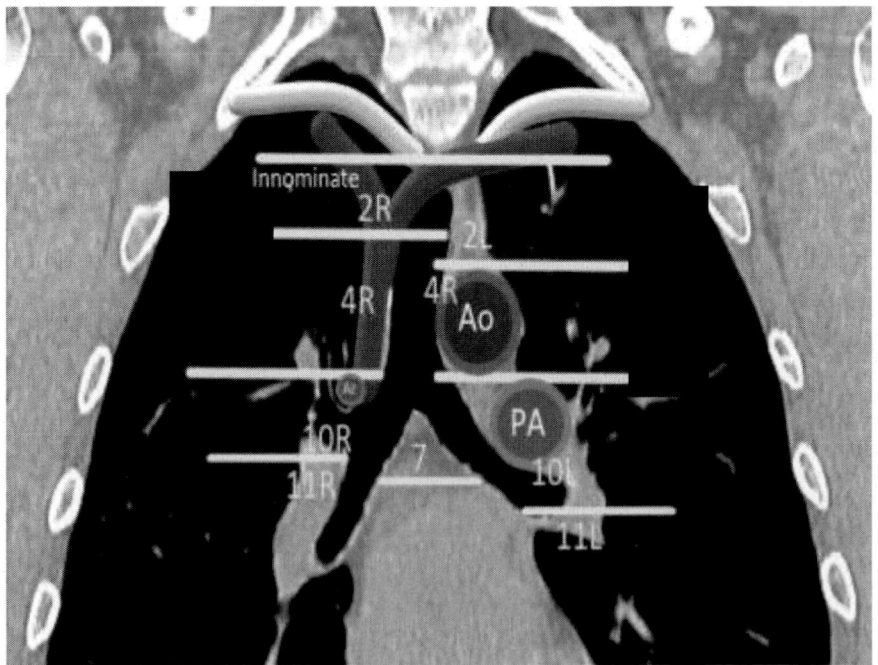

Figure 2. Mediastinal and hilar lymph node map of International Association for the Study of Lung Cancer (IASLC), reproduced with permission from IASLC.

MEDIASTINAL ADENOPATHY FROM EXTRATHORACIC METASTASIS

Many extrathoracic malignancies can invade into the thoracic cavity. Although these represent only a small portion of the usual pathologies causing mediastinal lymphadenopathy, they present complicated and serious diagnostic challenges. Extrathoracic malignancies known to invade the mediastinum are mainly breast cancer, head and neck tumors, gastrointestinal tumors, genitourinary tumors, renal cell carcinomas, and malignant melanomas. The exact incidence and prevalence of mediastinal and hilar metastasis from extrathoracic malignancies are relatively unknown.

One of the earliest studies investigating intrathoracic lymph node metastases from extrathoracic malignancies was conducted in the 1970s by McLoud and colleagues. They reviewed clinical records of 1,071 of extrathoracic malignancies and identified 25 (2.3%) cases with radiographic evidences of intrathoracic lymphadenopathies mainly via mediastinoscopy or surgical thoracotomy. Out of these 25 cases, 12 (48%) cases were associated with genitourinary malignancies, 8 (32%) from head and neck malignancies, 3 (12%) from breast malignancies, and 2 (8%) from melanomas. In their study, the most frequent location of the intrathoracic lymphadenopathy was right paratracheal lymph node group, followed by hilar lymph nodes [1]. This finding was reinforced by a case series of 50 cases with mediastinal and hilar lymphadenopathy with known infradiaphragmatic malignancies, revealing the most common location of a nodal involvement as the right paratracheal in 41 (82%) cases, subcarinal in 31 (62%), and hilar nodes in 21 (42%) cases [5].

More recent study utilizing data from 49 patients who underwent endoscopic ultrasound (EUS) guided fine needle aspiration (FNA) of isolated mediastinal and hilar lymphadenopathies with no known underlying malignancies, a metastatic malignancy of extrathoracic origin was identified in 14 of 49 cases (29%), malignant process of pulmonary origin in 4 cases (8%), benign process in 24 cases (49%), and non-diagnostic in 7 cases

(14%). Out of these cases, metastatic breast carcinoma was the most frequent at 6 of 14 (42.9%), followed by colon cancer (2 of 14, 14.3%), renal cell cancer (2 of 14, 14.3%), testicular cancer (2 of 14, 14.3%), esophageal cancer (1 of 14, 7.1%), and laryngeal cancer (1 of 14, 7.1%) [6]. This study only represents a single center experience with patients who specifically underwent EUS with fine needle aspiration as the choice of diagnostic procedure for reasons of feasibility and failure to obtain diagnosis via other available procedures. Nonetheless, the study highlighted a significant rate of metastatic invasion into the thoracic cavity by extrathoracic malignancies, particularly cancers from the breast, head and neck, gastrointestinal, and genitourinary origin (Figure 3). It also highlighted the possibility of mediastinal metastasis of lung cancer with no identifiable primary lung parenchymal lesion.

Table 1. Extrathoracic malignancies and the usual patterns of metastasis

Thoracic Lymph Nodes	Pulmonary Parenchyma	Both
Head and neck cancer	Bladder cancer	Breast cancer
Esophageal cancer	Neuroblastoma	Colon cancer
Hepatocellular cancer	Melanoma	Renal cell cancer
Thymic carcinoma	Sarcoma	Prostate cancer
	Wilm's tumor	

With the advent of endobronchial ultrasound-guided transbronchial needle aspiration (EBUS-TBNA) in investigation of thoracic lymphadenopathies, there has been more available data which supported similar findings [1]. In patients with known extrathoracic malignancy and concurrent mediastinal lymphadenopathy, the frequency of mediastinal nodal metastasis from extrathoracic malignancy was 43-52% [7,8,9]. Given the high prevalence of mediastinal invasion from metastatic cancer, prompt investigation including short interval CT scans, PET scans, and tissue biopsies are necessary. In addition, a new diagnosis of concurrent lung cancer was revealed in 12-22% of cases, again raising the importance of tissue sampling for histologic confirmation even in patients with a known primary cancer. It should be noted that some extrathoracic malignancies can also metastasize to the lung parenchyma in addition to mediastinal and hilar lymph nodes (Table 1).

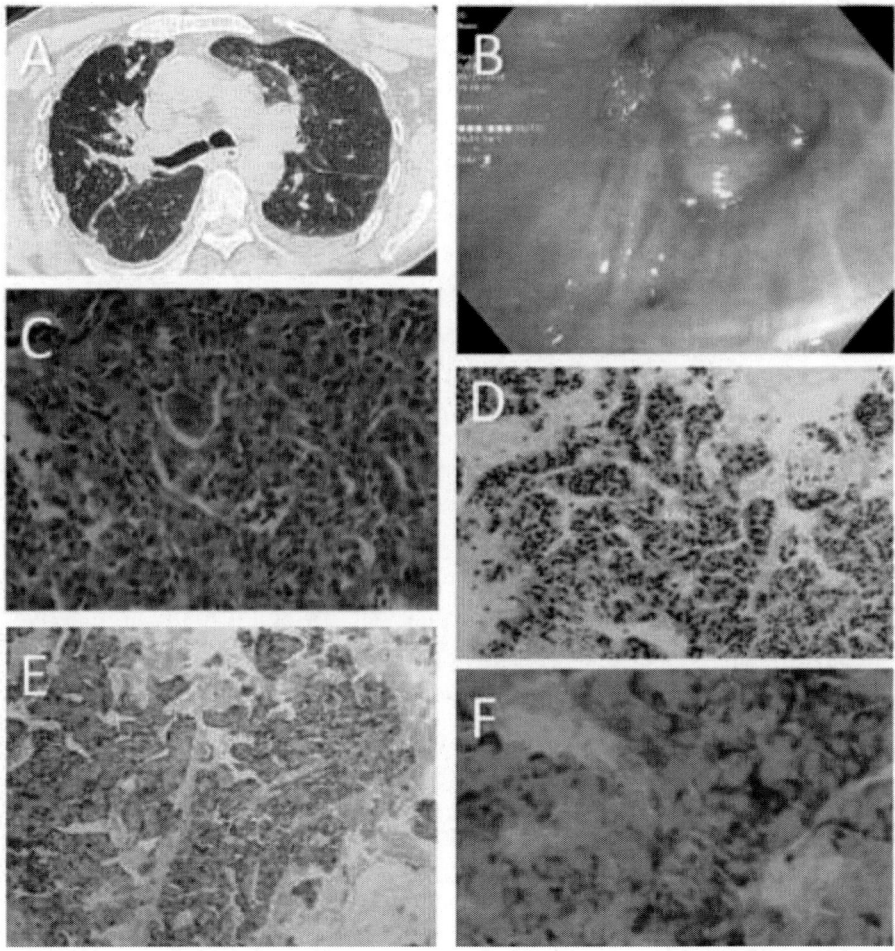

Figure 3 (A) Computed tomography scan of the chest highlighting right upper lobe obstruction with a soft tissue mass. (B) Bronchoscopic view of the polypoid endobronchial lesion in the right upper lobe bronchus. (C) The lung mass biopsy (H&E, x40) revealing infiltrating carcinoma with sheets of medium to large-sized carcinoma cells with abundant eosinophilic cytoplasm and prominent nucleoli. (D-F) Immunohistochemical stains on cell block show positive immunoreactivity for Androgen receptor (D, x20), PSA (E, x20) and AMACR (F, x40), consistent with metastatic carcinoma of prostate origin.

RADIOGRAPHIC SURVEILLANCE OF MEDIASTINAL ADENOPATHY

Mediastinal lymphadenopathies in setting of extrathoracic malignancies are usually detected by CT scans of the chest (Figure 4). Unlike the management and surveillance approaches for pulmonary nodules, there are no established guidelines for monitoring mediastinal and hilar lymphadenopathies in setting of potential metastatic process. The Fleischner Society guidelines, which provide the best-practice guidelines for pulmonary nodule surveillance, make it clear that the guideline is not intended to be used in patients with known primary cancers who are at risk for metastases [10]. Given that the rate of mediastinal and hilar lymph node metastasis in the setting of underlying extrathoracic malignancy approaches 50%, the need for comprehensive recommendations and guidelines is heightened.

Traditionally, mediastinal and hilar lymph nodes are considered abnormal if the short axis dimension is ≥ 10mm. This notion has been challenged in small studies such as a study by Evison and colleagues which suggested lymph nodes that were less than 15mm were virtually all reactive while any nodes greater than 25mm were more likely to be pathologic [11]. However it should be noted that there is no strict "cut-off" for the lymph node size that can be used to rule in or out any lymph nodes from its malignant potential.

In addition to size, other features of lymph nodes, such as shape, symmetry, density, texture, and presence of fatty hilum must all be considered in risk-stratifying the lymphadenopathy. Most benign nodes have smooth, well defined borders and have homogenous computed tomographic attenuation. The presence of central fatty hilum has been associated with benign causes of lymphadenopathy [12]. The symmetry seen in mediastinal lymphadenopathy provides helpful clues in forming differential diagnosis. The common causes of symmetrical lymphadenopathy include pneumoconiosis, amyloidosis, and Castleman's disease. Metastases are an uncommon cause of symmetrical disease, but this pattern is occasionally seen with gastrointestinal tumors, genitourinary tumors, lung cancers, breast cancers, and leukemias [13].

Lastly, the presence of calcification within the lymph node usually confers benign mineralization from granulomatous processes. However, calcification may also be associated with certain malignancies such as osteosarcoma, chondrosarcoma, papillary thyroid cancer, and mucinous tumors of gastrointestinal and genitourinary tracts [14]. With the increased utilization of EBUS and EUS, there has been an heightened interest in developing a scoring system to characterize mediastinal lymphadenopathy as benign versus malignant. From a recent study, Ayub and colleagues have found that the sonographic features of mediastinal lymph nodes that favor benign disease are well defined margins, presence of central hilar structure, and nodal conglomeration (Table 2). Among these features, the diagnostic accuracies for predicting benign nodal disease were highest for presence of well-defined margins and homogenous echogenicity (81.1% and 65.7% respectively) [15].

Given the rising prevalence of mediastinal and hilar lymphadenopathies due to the increased frequency of chest CT scans, the Incidental Findings Committee of the American College of Radiology (ACR) compiled its recommendations in 2018 based on the combination of current published evidence and expert opinion. The prevalence of incidental finding of mediastinal lymphadenopathy is estimated to be 1% to 6% [16,17]. The Committee recommends no further workup when an incidental mediastinal lymph node with a short axis diameter <15mm is found in an otherwise asymptomatic person with no other findings. If, however, the short axis diameter exceeds 15mm in asymptomatic person, further investigation is necessary. If there is no explainable disease such as underlying sarcoidosis, heart failure, or interstitial lung disease, then the ACR recommends a short-interval CT scan (3-6 months) or a positron emission tomography (PET) CT scan. A biopsy is recommended if there is an interval growth or clinical indication [14]. In general, if the lymphadenopathy is concurrent with an active infectious or inflammatory process, with no evidence of underlying malignancy, no further evaluation may be necessary.

PET scan uses fluorodeoxyglucose (FDG) as a tracer to assess metabolic activity of tissues and lymph nodes and can help differentiate normal tissues from diseased tissues. In setting of lung nodules, an FDG uptake of greater than 2.5 standardized uptake value (SUV) is widely accepted as the metabolic threshold to differentiate between malignant and benign pulmonary parenchymal lesions. Even in this setting, there are many infectious and inflammatory processes such as pulmonary sarcoidosis, rheumatoid nodules, tuberculosis, reactive lymphadenopathy, and endemic mycoses that can lead to false-positive results. On the other hand, malignant lesions such as carcinoid tumors, adenocarcinoma in situ, and smaller nodules with cross sectional diameter less than 10mm can lead to false-negative results in FDG-PET scans.

In the setting of isolated thoracic lymph adenopathy, the diagnosis becomes even more challenging and the utility of PET scan is less well defined. A study by Kumar and colleagues in 2011 reviewed FDG avidity of 35 patients with isolated thoracic lymphadenopathy without primary neoplasm or infectious lung pathologies who underwent PET scans. Benign causes had a significantly lower FDG uptake with a mean ± standard deviation (SD) of 5.02 ±3.26, compared to the FDG uptake of malignant causes which was 10.8 ±8.12. With SUVmax of 2.5, the sensitivity was 93% with specificity of 40% to discriminate between malignant and benign lymph nodes in this study. The authors highlighted poor specificity, positive predictive value, and diagnostic accuracy of FDG-PET scans, especially in an area with high prevalence of thoracic granulomatous diseases [18].

In general, if there is a finding of mediastinal or hilar lymphadenopathy in patient with known cancer, a multidisciplinary approach involving medical and surgical oncologists, radiologists, interventional radiologists, radiation oncologists, interventional pulmonologists, and palliative care specialists should be undertaken to discuss feasible biopsy options and review available treatment approaches. Although past studies showed 50% rate of metastatic process in this setting, the possibilities of primary lung cancer, concurrent infectious or inflammatory processes, and benign etiologies should be considered.

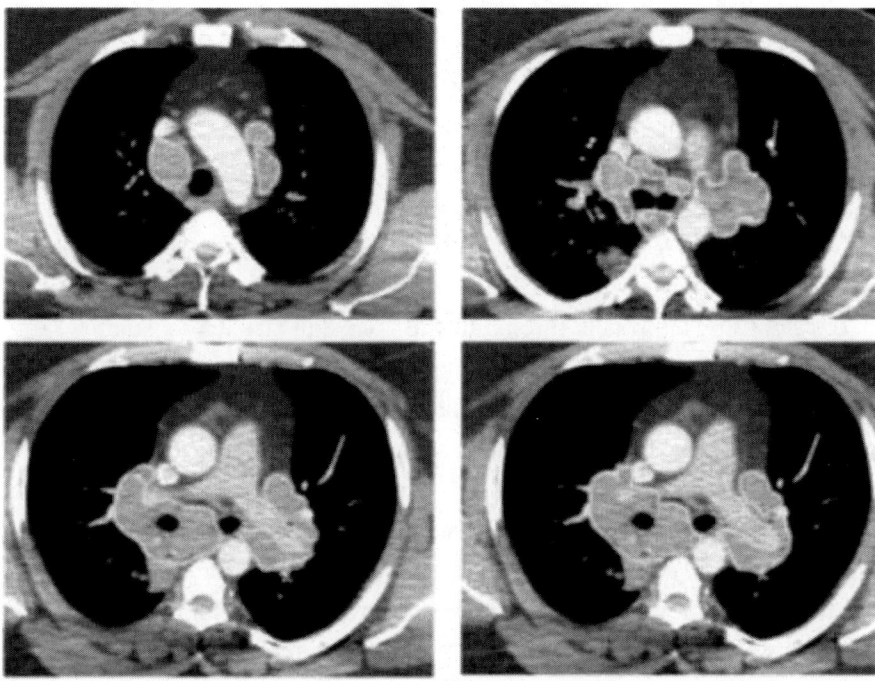

Figure 4. CT scan of a patient with extensive mediastinal and hilar lymphadenopathy.

Table 2. Radiographic and sonographic features of benign versus malignant disease

Benign	Malignant
Symmetric distribution (Pneumoconiosis, amyloidosis, Castleman's disease)	Asymmetric distribution (Most of metastatic malignancies and lymphomas follow this pattern)
Presence of fatty hilum	Larger size
Homogenous attenuation	Heterogeneous attenuation
Calcification of lymph nodes	
Distinct margin	
Presence of central hilar structures (a linear, flat, hyper-echoic area in the center of lymph node)	
Nodal conglomeration	

DIAGNOSTIC STEPS

There are several invasive methods to sample mediastinal and hilar lymph nodes, which include esophageal ultrasound (EUS), endobronchial ultrasound (EBUS), mediastinoscopy, and video-assisted thoracic surgery (VATS) (Figure 5). Prior to the advent of minimally invasive sampling methods, such as EUS and EBUS, mediastinoscopy was the most widely utilized sampling approach. It remains the gold standard diagnostic modality for mediastinal lymphadenopathies, however it requires general anesthesia and has 2% morbidity rate [19]. Mediastinoscopy's diagnostic sensitivity in setting of extrathoracic malignancy is variable and uncertain. It does not allow access to the inferior and posterior mediastinum, hilum, and interlobar nodes. There are two additional settings that make mediastinoscopy disadvantageous: cases that require a repeat mediastinoscopy, and for patients who underwent radiation therapy to the thorax. A repeat mediastinoscopy can be significantly more challenging with the adhesions from the first operation, and fibrotic changes from radiation can make the anatomy less amenable for proper tissue sampling [20]. Recently, EBUS has become an initial method for biopsying mediastinal region as it allows access to paratracheal, subcarinal, and hilar lymph node stations bilaterally whereas EUS does not allow access to right paratracheal and hilar stations, limiting its use in staging of malignancies. Furthermore, mediastinoscopy cannot evaluate the hilar lymph nodes, which can be the sole area with a significant lymphadenopathy [20, 21]. For lung cancer diagnosis and staging, EBUS has been established to have a sensitivity that is greater than 90%. The data on EBUS and its performance on diagnosis in setting of extrathoracic cancers is not as robust, but recent studies have reported overall sensitivity, accuracy, negative predictive value of EBUS with transbronchial needle aspiration (TBNA) as 87-90%, 88-96%, and 73-93% respectively (Figure 6) [7,22,23]. EBUS is a very safe procedure, with complications that include airway irritation, bleeding, and pneumothorax. Risk of pneumothorax with EBUS alone is 0.2% and increases to 2.7% when transbronchial biopsy is performed in conjunction [24]. Also repeat EBUS procedures are just as safe as the initial EBUS given the lack of anatomic distortion caused by the procedure itself. Combining its high diagnostic accuracy and sensitivity with low serious complication rates, EBUS is a promising minimally invasive outpatient procedure in investigating mediastinal and hilar lymphadenopathy.

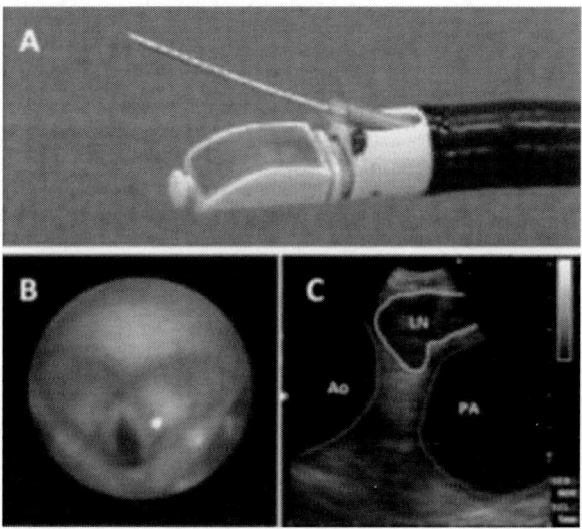

Figure 5. (A) Convex EBUS probe with the biopsy needle (B) The 30-degree forward oblique view of the vocal cord using the EBUS bronchoscope (C) Lymph node station 4L between the aorta and pulmonary artery.

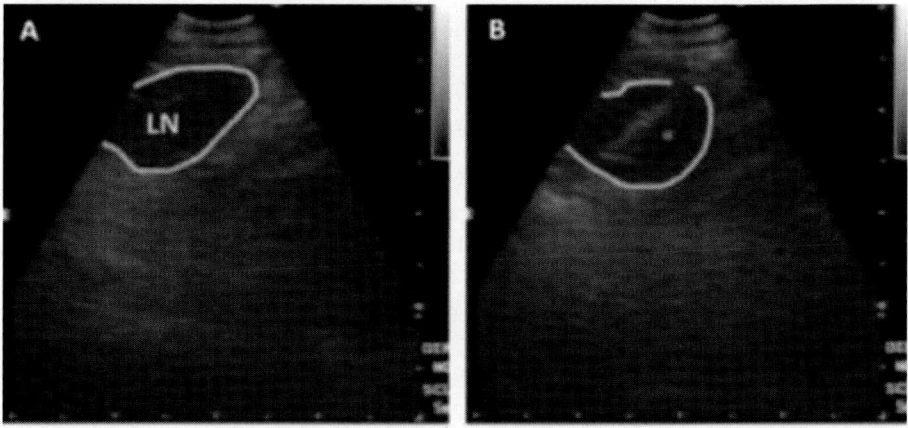

Figure 6. (A) Endobronchial ultrasound view of a lymph node (B) Transbronchial needle in the lymph node shown with an asterisk.

IMMUNOHISTOCHEMICAL STAINING IN EXTRATHORACIC MALIGNANCIES

Immunohistochemical staining is performed to assess the histological origin of the samples obtained through EBUS-TBNA. This becomes increasingly significant in cases of undiagnosed mediastinal lymphadenopathy, in particular with increase in the number of cytological samples being obtained through minimally invasive procedures.

Tumors with clear morphologic patterns can be diagnosed with limited immunohistochemical markers of pneumocyte origin including TTF-1 for adenocarcinoma and p40 for squamous cell carcinoma. Napsin A is also an acceptable marker of adenocarcinoma differentiation, although less readily available in some areas. Similarly, Cytokeratin 5/6 are acceptable markers of squamous cell differentiation. If both morphologic patterns are present in the sample and confirmed by histologic markers, a diagnosis of adenosquamous carcinoma is possible but can only be confirmed on resected samples. Pulmonary small cell carcinomas express TTF-1 with variable chromogranin and synaptophysin staining (Table 3). In cases of non-small cell carcinoma which do not express histological markers of pneumocyte origin, further evaluation is warranted to determine the primary site.

Table 3. Immunohistochemical stains for lung cancer

Histologic Subtype	Immunohistochemical Stain
Adenocarcinoma	TTF-1 CK-7 NAPSIN
Squamous Cell Cancer	CK-5 CK-6 P-40
Small Cell Cancer	TTF-1 SYNAPTOPHYSIN CHROMOGRANIN

Histologic adenocarcinomas with negative pneumocyte immunehistologic markers, CK-7 and CK-20 stains can be used to identify tumors of GI origin which only express CK-20 reactivity in contrast to their pulmonary counterparts that only express CK-7 reactivity. Pancreatic adenocarcinomas however express both CK-7 and variable CK-20 reactivity but is CA-199 positive. Similarly, tumors of prostate origin express PSA reactivity with negative CK-7 and CK20 stains. Metastatic tumors from other primary sites including breast, renal, uroepithelial and ovarian cancers can be diagnosed by their distinct morphology and tumor markers including ER, PR, Her-2-Neu, CEA, WT1 and CA-125 (Table 4) [25]. Similarly, molecular testing has become increasingly significant with the wide array of available targeted immune therapies. At present, testing for ALK, EGFR and PD-L1 is recommended by current oncology guidelines on NSCLC samples and NSCC NOS [26].

Table 4. Immunohistochemical stains for metastatic cancer

TUMOR TYPE	POSITIVE	NEGATIVE
Colorectal Cancer	CK-20	CK-7
Hepatocellular Cancer	CEA AFP HEP PAR 1	CK-7 CK-20
Pancreatic Cancer	CA-199 CK-7	
Renal Cell Cancer	CK-7 VIMENTIN Pan Keratin	CK-20 CEA
Breast Cancer	ER PR Her-2-Neu GATA-3	CK-20
Ovarian Cancer	CK-7 ER WT-1	CK-20
Neuroendocrine Cancer	CHROMOGRANIN SYNAPTOPHYSIN	
Germ Cell Tumor	HCG AFP	

CONCLUSION

Although mediastinal or hilar lymph node metastases of extrathoracic malignancies are observed in varying frequencies, they are not as widespread as lung cancer. Many extrathoracic malignancies can metastasize to lungs, mediastinal, and hilar lymph nodes. The main types of cancer that are known to invade the thoracic lymph node are breast cancer, head and neck cancer, colorectal cancer, genitourinary cancer, renal cell carcinoma, and malignant melanoma. In patients with extrapulmonary malignancy, mediastinal and hilar lymph node enlargement may also be due to tuberculosis, granulomatous inflammation, and reactive changes. If these mediastinal lesions are found to be metastasis, then the staging, prognosis, and treatment strategies change dramatically for these patients, thus a multidisciplinary approach that aligns with patients' goals of care should be utilized. CT scans and PET scans are imaging methods that are frequently used in the evaluation of mediastinal or hilar lesions. However, these methods cannot make the distinction between malignant and benign lesions and cannot ensure the pathological confirmation. Therefore, cytopathological sampling is required in these cases. Previously, surgical methods were widely applied in the evaluation of mediastinal lymphadenopathies in cases with extrathoracic malignancy. However, less invasive methods such as EBUS are used instead of surgical methods. EBUS-TBNA is a highly sensitive modality for the diagnosis of mediastinal and hilar metastasis from extrapulmonary malignancy and can be considered as an initial test for the histopathological diagnosis.

REFERENCES

[1] McLoud, T. C., Kalisher, L., Stark, P., Greene, R. *Intrathoracic lymph node metastases from extrathoracic neoplasms.* AJR Am J Roentgenol. 1978;131(3):403-407.

[2] Naruke, T., Suemasu, K., Ishikawa, S. *Lymph node mapping and curability at various levels of metastasis in resected lung cancer.* J Thorac Cardiovasc Surg. 1978;76(6):832-839.

[3] Mountain, C. F., Dresler, C. M. *Regional lymph node classification for lung cancer staging.* Chest. 1997;111(6):1718-1723.

[4] El-Sherief, A. H., Lau, C. T., Wu, C. C., Drake, R. L., Abbott, G. F., Rice, T. W. *International Association for the Study of Lung Cancer (IASLC) Lymph Node Map: Radiologic Review with CT Illustration.* RadioGraphics. 2014;34(6):1680-1691.

[5] Mahon, T. G., Libshitz, H. I. *Mediastinal metastases of infradiaphragmatic malignancies.* Eur J Radiol. 1992;15(2):130-134.

[6] Devereaux, B. M., LeBlanc, J. K., Yousif, E., et al. *Clinical utility of EUS-guided fine-needle aspiration of mediastinal masses in the absence of known pulmonary malignancy.* Gastrointestinal Endoscopy. 2002;56(3):397-401.

[7] Navani, N., Nankivell, M., Woolhouse, I., et al. *Endobronchial ultrasound-guided transbronchial needle aspiration for the diagnosis of intrathoracic lymphadenopathy in patients with extrathoracic malignancy: a multicenter study.* J Thorac Oncol. 2011;6(9):1505-1509.

[8] Sanz-Santos, J., Cirauqui, B., Sanchez, E., et al. *Endobronchial ultrasound-guided transbronchial needle aspiration in the diagnosis of intrathoracic lymph node metastases from extrathoracic malignancies.* Clinical & Experimental Metastasis. 2013;30(4):521-528.

[9] Chaddha, U., Patil, P. D., English, R., Panchabhai, T. S. *An Unusual Presentation of Cervical Carcinoma Metastasis as Mediastinal Adenopathy.* J Bronchology Interv Pulmonol. 2017;24(4):e61-e63.

[10] MacMahon, H., Naidich, D. P., Goo, J. M., et al. *Guidelines for Management of Incidental Pulmonary Nodules Detected on CT Images: From the Fleischner Society 2017.* Radiology. 2017;284(1):228-243.

[11] Evison, M., Crosbie, P. A. J., Morris, J., Martin, J., Barber, P. V., Booton, R. *A study of patients with isolated mediastinal and hilar*

lymphadenopathy undergoing EBUS-TBNA. BMJ Open Respiratory Research. 2014;1(1):e000040.

[12] Torabi, M., Aquino, S. L., Harisinghani, M. G. *Current concepts in lymph node imaging.* J Nucl Med. 2004;45(9):1509-1518.

[13] Elicker, B., Webb, W. *Fundamentals of High-Resolution Lung CT: Common Findings, Common Patterns, Common Diseases, and Differential Diagnosis.* Wolters Kluwer; 2013.

[14] Munden, R. F., Carter, B. W., Chiles, C., et al. *Managing Incidental Findings on Thoracic CT: Mediastinal and Cardiovascular Findings. A White Paper of the ACR Incidental Findings Committee.* J Am Coll Radiol. 2018;15(8):1087-1096.

[15] Ayub, II, Mohan, A., Madan, K., et al. Identification of specific EBUS sonographic characteristics for predicting benign mediastinal lymph nodes. *The Clinical Respiratory Journal.* 2018;12(2):681-690.

[16] Gil, B. N., Ran, K., Tamar, G., Shmuell, F., Eli, A. *Prevalence of significant noncardiac findings on coronary multidetector computed tomography angiography in asymptomatic patients.* J Comput Assist Tomogr. 2007;31(1):1-4.

[17] Jacobs, P. C. A., Mali, W. P. T. M., Grobbee, D. E., van der Graaf, Y. *Prevalence of incidental findings in computed tomographic screening of the chest: a systematic review.* J Comput Assist Tomogr. 2008;32(2):214-221.

[18] Kumar, A., Dutta, R., Kannan, U., Kumar, R., Khilnani, G. C., Gupta, S. D. *Evaluation of mediastinal lymph nodes using F-FDG PET-CT scan and its histopathologic correlation.* Ann Thorac Med. 2011;6(1):11-16.

[19] Detterbeck, F. C., Jantz, M. A., Wallace, M., Vansteenkiste, J., Silvestri, G. A., *American College of Chest Physicians. Invasive mediastinal staging of lung cancer: ACCP evidence-based clinical practice guidelines (2nd edition).* Chest. 2007;132(3 Suppl):202S-220S.

[20] Yasufuku, K., Nakajima, T., Fujiwara, T., et al. *Role of endobronchial ultrasound-guided transbronchial needle aspiration in the*

management of lung cancer. Gen Thorac Cardiovasc Surg. 2008;56(6):268-276.

[21] Kim, H., Kadura, S., Safi, J., Singh, H., Khemasuwan, D. *EBUS Basics and Mediastinal Staging. American Thoracic Society, Best of ATS* Video Lecture Series; 2019. https://www.thoracic.org/professionals/clinical-resources/video-lecture-series/bronchoscopy/ebus-basics-and-mediastinal-staging.php.

[22] Song, J-U., Yun Park, H., Jeon, K., et al. *The Role of Endobronchial Ultrasound-Guided Transbronchial Needle Aspiration in the Diagnosis of Mediastinal and Hilar Lymph Node Metastases in Patients with Extrapulmonary Malignancy.* Internal Medicine. 2011;50(21):2525-2532.

[23] Tertemiz, K. C., Alpaydin, A. O., Karacam, V. *The role of endobronchial ultrasonography for mediastinal lymphadenopathy in cases with extrathoracic malignancy.* Surgical Endoscopy. 2017;31(7):2829-2836.

[24] Eapen, G. A., Shah, A. M., Lei, X., et al. *Complications, consequences, and practice patterns of endobronchial ultrasound-guided transbronchial needle aspiration: Results of the AQuIRE registry.* Chest. 2013;143(4):1044-1053.

[25] Travis, W. D., *Weltgesundheitsorganisation, International Agency for Research on Cancer,* eds. WHO Classification of Tumours of Lung, Pleura, Thymus and Heart: ... Reflects the Views of a Working Group That Convened for a Consensus and Editorial Meeting at the International Agency for Research on Cancer, Lyon, April 24 - 26, 2014. 4. ed. Lyon: International Agency for Research on Cancer; 2015.

[26] Thunnissen, E., Kerr, K. M., Herth, F. J. F., et al. *The challenge of NSCLC diagnosis and predictive analysis on small samples.* Practical approach of a working group. Lung Cancer. 2012;76(1):1-18.

In: Thoracic Lymphadenopathy
Editor: Vikas Pathak

ISBN: 978-1-53616-700-9
© 2020 Nova Science Publishers, Inc.

Chapter 4

LYMPHOMA

Santosh Nepal, MD
Geisinger Holy Spirit Hospital, Camp Hill, Pennsylvania, US

INTRODUCTION

Mediastinum is a complex anatomical structure and is involved in multitude of diseases, some primary affecting it while other spreading from other organs. Lymph node in the mediastinum and bilateral hila can be involved in infective, inflammatory or malignant process. Malignancy can be a metastatic lesion or a primary involvement. Lymphoma is one of the important differential diagnosis of the mediastinal and hilar lymphadenopathy as this account for 20% of primary mediastinal tumor in adults [1].

Thorax, mainly in the form of mediastinal or hilar lymphadenopathy is involved in 85% of all cases of Hodgkin's Lymphoma (HL) where as 45% of all cases of Non-Hodgkin's Lymphoma [2, 3]. It is very important to consider other possible diagnosis for mediastinal and Hilar lymphadenopathy as these can frequently be infective or inflammatory with a completely different treatment strategy. Although certain radiological characteristics indicate lymphoma, biopsy is the definite way to diagnose.

LYMPHOMA

Lymphoma is broadly divided into Hodgkin's Lymphoma (HL) and Non-Hodgkin's Lymphoma (NHL). NHL is more common and represents nearly 85% of lymphomas [4].

NHL can be aggressive or indolent. Diffuse Large B Cell Lymphoma (DLBCL) is the most common and aggressive NHL, followed by Mantle Cell lymphoma (MCL) and adult T-cell Leukemia/lymphoma. Indolent lymphoma has better prognosis and consists of Follicular Lymphoma (FL), Marginal Zone Lymphoma (MZL) and Small-Cell Lymphocytic Lymphoma (SCLL). Based on histological characteristics and tumor cell phenotype, HL is subdivided into the classical and non-classical types. Classical type comprises of four histological subtypes -Nodular Sclerosis, Lymphocyte Predominance, Mixed Cellularity and Lymphocytic Depletion.

Non-classical type includes the Nodular lymphocyte predominant type [5].

IMAGING IN LYMPHOMA

Although Chest x-ray may show some indication of hilar or mediastinal lymphadenopathy, contrast enhanced CT of the chest provides detailed evaluation. Some of the suggestive characteristics for lymphoma include:

1) Coalescence of Lymphadenopathy: This is significantly higher in lymphoma (up to 94.6% in Hodgkin's lymphoma) compared to 5.3% in Sarcoid [6].

2) Calcification: Very rarely present in lymphoma although this can be seen after treatment (2.7% in Lymphoma versus 30.8 in Sarcoid) [7].
3) Anatomical distortion: Seen in lymphoma (59.5%) in Hodgkin's lymphoma and none in Sarcoid [6].
4) Site of involvement: Mediastinal lymph node without hilar lymph node is more suggestive of lymphoma whereas bilateral hilar lymphadenopathy without mediastinal lymph node is more suggestive for granulomatous disease like Sarcoid. Similarly, if we see unilateral hilar lymphadenopathy, the chance of it being Lymphoma is more than Sarcoid (37.8% vs less than 8%). Upper para-tracheal, pre-vascular and pre-tracheal region are more commonly involved in HL. Anterior mediastinum and para-tracheal region tend to be more involved along with contiguous spread in HL [8].
5) Pattern of enhancement may also help in differential. Lymphoma tends to be of homogenous enhancement (83% both HL and NHL in one series) [9]. The lymphadenopathy is not overtly hyper vascular. When hypervascularity is present alternative diagnosis including Carcinoid, Castleman's disease, para-ganglioma, vascular malformation and nodal metastasis from other primary malignancy [10].

ROLE OF FUNCTIONAL IMAGING

Although gallium scan has been used in the past. PET scan is currently in widespread use with better sensitivity in detecting the nodal involvement along with extra-nodal lesions including the splenic lesions and bone marrow involvement [11]. It plays an important role in staging, restaging, prognostication, planning appropriate treatment strategies, monitoring therapy, and detecting recurrence. The data on this is, however, mostly retrospective. In one retrospective study with 172 patients with suspected lymphoma at the University of Pennsylvania, FDG-PET detected disease in at least one site in 161 patients (94%) and failed to detect disease in 11 patients (6%). FDG-PET detected disease in 100% of patients with Large B Cell Lymphoma and Marginal Zone Lymphoma and in 98% of patients with Hodgkin's Lymphoma and Follicular Lymphoma. In contrast, FDG-PET detected disease in only 67% of Mantle Zone Lymphoma and 40% of Peripheral T Cell Lymphoma [12].

DIAGNOSIS

Biopsy is the definite diagnostic test for Lymphoma. Although mediastinoscopy is a gold standard for obtaining a sample from these lymph nodes, not all regions are accessible, including sub-carinal and infra-hilar lymph nodes. Besides, mediastinoscopy is costly, requires patient to be admitted and is more invasive. Trans Bronchial Needle Aspiration (TBNA) is a minimally invasive method to obtain the sample, however its sensitivity varied between 25 - 85% in the past depending on the location and size of the node. Introduction of Endo-Bronchial Ultrasound (EBUS) for TBNA has significantly increased the diagnostic yield.

The study looking at the usefulness of aspiration biopsy through EBUS are largely retrospective and has varying results. In one of such study by Erer et al. [13] when a series of 13 diagnosed cases of Lymphoma were included, none of the Hodgkin lymphoma (HL) cases could be diagnosed with EBUS-TBNA. The overall diagnostic sensitivity and NPV of EBUS-TBNA in detecting lymphoma was 65% and 96.1%, respectively. For the newly diagnosed lymphoma cases, EBUS-TBNA had a sensitivity of 61.1%.

It is important to note that current diagnostic modality not only include cyto-morphology but also cyto-genetics, immuno-phenotyping and molecular markers thus increasing the diagnostic accuracy even with the smaller samples, increasing the diagnostic sensitivity.

Although Americal College of Chest Physicians recommends EBUS TBNA as an initial diagnostic modality to get samples from mediastinal and hilar lymphadenopathy [14], NCCN (National Comprehensive Cancer Network) recommends avoiding this as an initial diagnosis unless for the evaluation of recurrent Lymphoma [15, 16]. European Society of Medical Oncology (ESMO) recommends larger samples but did not specify the modalities [17].

Overall, with proper patient counseling about the possibility of an inconclusive result, EBUS TBNA can definitely be an initial modality for diagnosis. Not only can it aid on diagnosis but will also help diagnose alternative cause for mediastinal and hilar lymphadenopathy.

SUMMARY

Lymphoma is one of the important and common causes of mediastinal and hilar lymphadenopathy. There are certain imaging characteristic and anatomic predilection, which may aid in the diagnosis of Lymphoma. Tissue biopsy remains the cornerstone for diagnosis although the modality to obtain the sample may differ. Less invasive modalities like EBUS TBNA can be of immense help if performed and analyzed in the proper clinical setting without the need for more invasive procedure like mediastinoscopy.

REFERENCES

[1] Takahashi, K., Al-Janabi, N. J. Computed tomography and magnetic resonance imaging of mediastinal tumors. *J. Magn. Reson. Imaging,* 2010 Dec.; 32(6):1325 - 39.

[2] El-Sherief, A. H., Lau, C. T., Wu et al. (2014). International Association for the Study of Lung Cancer (IASLC) Lymph Node Map: Radiologic Review with CT Illustration. *Radiographics*, 2014. 34(6), 1680 - 1691.

[3] Bligh, M. P., Borgaonkar, J. N., Burrell et al. Spectrum of CT Findings in Thoracic Extranodal Non-Hodgkin Lymphoma. *Radiographics,* 2017; 37(2):439 - 461.

[4] Lu, P. Staging and classification of lymphoma. *Semin. Nucl. Med.,* 2005; 35:160 - 164.

[5] Küppers, R., Engert, A., Hansmann, M. L. *J. Clin. Invest.,* 2012 Oct; 122(10):3439 - 47.

[6] Mehrian P, Ebrahimzadeh SA. Differentiation between sarcoidosis and Hodgkin's lymphoma based on mediastinal lymph node involvement pattern: Evaluation using spiral CT scan. Pol J Radiol. 2013 Jul;78(3):15-20.

[7] Panicek, D. M., Harty, M. P., Scicutella, C. J. et al. Calcification in untreated mediastinal lymphoma. *Radiology,* 1988; 166:735 - 6.

[8] Sharma, A., Fidias, P., Hayman, L. A. et al. Patterns of lymphadenopathy in thoracic malignancies. *Radiographics,* 2004; 24:419 - 34.

[9] Tang, S.S. et al. Differentiation between tuberculosis and lymphoma in mediastinal lymph nodes: Evaluation with contrast-enhanced MDCT. *Clinical Radiology,* Volume 67, Issue 9, 877 - 883.

[10] Li, S. M., Hsu, H. H., Lee, S. C. et al. Mediastinal hemangioma presenting a characteristic feature on dynamic computed tomography images. *J. Thorac Dis.,* 2017; 9:E412 - 5.

[11] Ngeow, J. Y., Quek, R. H., Ng, D. C. et al. High SUV uptake on FDG-PET/CT predicts for an aggressive B-cell lymphoma in a prospective study of primary FDG-PET/CT staging in lymphoma. *Ann Oncol.,* 2009 Sep; 20(9):1543-7.

[12] Elstrom, R., Guan, L., Baker, G. et al. Utility of FDG-PET scanning in lymphoma by WHO classification. *Blood*, 2003; 101:3875 - 3876.

[13] Erer, O. F., Erol, S., Anar, C. et al. Diagnostic yield of EBUS-TBNA for lymphoma and review of the literature. *Endosc. Ultrasound,* 2017 Sep.-Oct.; 6(5):317 - 322.

[14] Wahidi, M. M., Herth, F., Yasufuku, K. et al. Technical aspects of endobronchial ultrasound-guided transbronchial needle aspiration: CHEST guideline and expert panel report. *Chest,* 2016; 149:816 - 835.

[15] Zelenetz, A. D., Gordon, L. I., Wierda, W. G. et al. Non-Hodgkin's lymphomas. *J. Natl. Compr. Canc. Netw.,* 2014; 12: 1282 - 1303.

[16] Hoppe, R., Advani, R., Ai, W. et al. Hodgkin lymphoma. *NCCN Clinical Practice Guideline*: 2014.

[17] Eichenauer, D. A., Engert, A., Andre, M. et al. Hodgkin's lymphoma: ESMO Clinical Practice Guidelines for diagnosis, treatment and follow-up. *Ann. Oncol.,* 2014.

In: Thoracic Lymphadenopathy
Editor: Vikas Pathak

ISBN: 978-1-53616-700-9
© 2020 Nova Science Publishers, Inc.

Chapter 5

INFECTIOUS DISEASES

Fahad Gul[1], MD and Abesh Niroula[2], MD
[1]Albert Einstein Healthcare Network, Philadelphia, Pennyslvania, US
[2]Emory University School of Medicine, Atlanta, Georgia, US

INTRODUCTION

Hilar and mediastinal lymphadenopathy can represent malignant, inflammatory, and infectious pathologies. Benign versus malignant etiologies can be difficult to differentiate given the indolent nature of malignancies and of primary pulmonary infections associated with mediastinal and hilar lymphadenopathy. Radiographic characteristics unique to pulmonary infections can be used in context of their clinical presentation and laboratory evaluation to aid in prompt diagnosis and treatment. The aim of this chapter will be to focus on infectious etiologies with known thoracic lymphadenopathy and their radiographic features, diagnostic evaluation, and treatment strategies.

DIAGNOSIS

Definition

Lymphadenopathy is defined as abnormalities in lymph node size, density, and number [1]. Common causes of hilar and mediastinal lymphadenopathy include malignancies, systemic inflammatory causes and several intrapulmonary infections. Defining key features of nodal disease can be useful in differentiating malignant from benign disease.

Size and Location

Normal lymph node size is determined by measurement along the lymph node's short axis (<1 cm) and regional location within the thorax [2-3]. Computed tomography (CT) is a useful imaging modality in determining lymph node number, size, architecture [4]. Long-axis measurements are not reliable due to their dependence on spatial orientation of the nodes. Short-axis measurements can also be distorted due to variable nodal orientation but with less error compared to long-axis measurements.

Shape and Texture

Shape and texture analysis on CT can accurately differentiate benign from malignant causes. Malignant lymph nodes have a heterogeneous appearance with a round shape, irregular boarders and varied contrast enhancement. Benign lymphadenopathy etiologies, including TB and fungal infections, have an elongated shape, central hypo density, and presence of perinodal fat [6].

DIFFERENTIAL DIAGNOSIS

Tuberculosis

Tuberculosis (TB) is an airborne infection caused by mycobacterium tuberculosis. Inhalation of aerosolized droplets of TB can lead to one of four following outcomes: immediate organism clearance, primary infection with active pulmonary disease, latent infection, and reactivation disease.

The initial focus of pulmonary infection is referred to as a Ghon focus. On chest radiographs it is usually found in the mid to lower right lung zones due to the inhalation pattern of the particles [8]. These Ghon foci will represent small areas of granulomatous changes that may appear on radiographs if enlarging or demonstrating areas of calcification. Lymphatic and hematogenous spread of the organism to adjacent lymph node results in the formation of a Gohn complex. Fibrosis and calcification of this complex leads to the development of a Ranke complex [8].

Lymphadenopathy is the most commonly observed feature on chest radiographs of patients afflicted with primary TB. On CT scan lymph nodes can have a heterogeneous enhancement with a central hypo density representing caseous necrosis and a hyper dense outer rim secondary to reactive granulomatous inflammation [9]. Unilateral airspace consolidation may also be seen on chest X-ray in 70% of children with primary TB. CT scan typically demonstrates homogenous consolidation but may also be patchy, linear, or nodular. Pleural effusions are also seen, usually unilateral and on the same side as the primary TB focus [10].

Reactivation TB appears as patchy and heterogeneous consolidation involving the upper lobes. 20-45% of patients will have cavitation present. Only 5 to 10% of patients with reactivation TB will have hilar and mediastinal lymphadenopathy [10]. CT scan by comparison is more sensitive for subtle localized disease and mediastinal and hilar lymphadenopathy [11].

Fungal Infections

Fungal infections including histoplasmosis and coccidiodomycosis and rarely blastomycosis can cause intrathoracic lymphadenopathy. Histoplasma capsulatum is the most common endemic mycosis in the United States and causes pulmonary infection through inhalation of spores from bird and bat droppings [12]. Similar to TB, the acute infection of histoplasmosis can lead to development of intrathoracic lymphadenopathy [13]. Once in the alveoli, neutrophils and macrophages phagocytize the organism but are unable to kill it. This leads to hematogenous spread of the organism and development of regional lymphadenopathy [14]. This can lead to development of a mediastinal granuloma with enlarged caseous lymph nodes that can result in fibrosing mediastinitis [16].

On chest X-ray hilar or mediastinal lymph adenopathy will usually be seen but may also be normal in the setting of acute infection. This adenopathy may persist for years with calcifications developing over time [15]. Chronic pulmonary histoplamosis can radiographically appear similar to reactivation TB with fibrotic apical infiltrates and cavitations present on chest X-ray and CT scan. Also, like reactivation TB, hilar and mediastinal lymphadenopathy is uncommonly seen in chronic infection [17].

Coccidioidomycoses is another dimorphic fungus endemic to the southwestern region of the United States that is contracted by inhalation of spores through the respiratory tract. Acute pulmonary infection results in parenchymal abnormalities with associated hilar and or mediastinal lymphadenopathy in 40% [18]. Lymph node abnormalities may persist for years after initial onset of infection.

Viral Infections

Varicella-zoster virus (VZV), measles virus, Epstein-Barr Virus (EBV), influenza virus can cause lower respiratory tract infection with radiological manifestations including consolidation, nodules, ground-glass opacification, and uncommonly thoracic lymphadenopathy.

Table 1. Differential Diagnosis of Infectious Thoracic Lymphadenopathy and associated clinical and radiographic features and treatment

	Clinical Presentation	Radiographic Features	Treatment
Latent Tuberculosis	90% asymptomatic. Initial infection may present with fever, shortness of breath, productive cough, erythema nodosum	Gohn focus or Gohn complex. Hilar and mediastinal lymphadenopathy	Isoniazid alone for 6 to 9 months or rifampin alone for 4 months or rifampin plus isoniazid for 3 months or rifapentine and isoniazid for 3 months
Active Tuberculosis	Chronic cough, sputum production, appetite loss, weight loss, fever, night sweats, hemoptysis	Upper airway cavitations, heterogeneous consolidation, rare hilar and mediastinal lymphadenopathy	Non-Multi Drug Resistant: Isoniazid, rifampin, ethambutol, pyrazinamide for 2 months and then isoniazid and rifampin for 4 months. Multi Drug Resistant: Four second line TB agents
Histoplasmosis	Acute infection: majority asymptomatic, may present with fever, fatigue, hepatosplenomegaly, pancytopenia. Chronic infection: Hepatosplenomegaly, pancytopenia, skin, brain, gastrointestinal involvement	Hilar and mediastinal lymphadenopathy. Calcifications may be seen. Cavitations, heterogeneous consolidation with chronic infection	Moderate to severe pulmonary disease: Amphotericin B for 1 to 2 weeks followed by itraconazole for 12 weeks. Mild pulmonary disease: Symptoms less than 4 weeks require no treatment, symptoms over 4 weeks can be treated with itraconazole for 6 to 12 weeks.
Coccidiodomycosis	Majority of infections are subclinical, may present initially with Fever, chest pain, cough, dyspnea. Severe disease can present with weight loss, night sweats, and rheumatologic and dermatologic manifestations	Hilar and mediastinal lymphadenopathy that may persist for years after initial infection. Uncommon Para pneumonic effusions, nodules, and cavitary formations.	Mild disease: Does not require treatment. Moderate to severe disease: Fluconazole or itraconazole for 3 to 6 months. Amphotericin B reserved for the most severe cases.
Viral Infections	Dependent on underlying viral etiology	Bilateral hilar and medistinal lymphadenopathy	Symptomatic management

EBV is most commonly associated with lymphadenopathy development. Case reports have demonstrated bilateral hilar and mediastinal lymphadenopathy associated with acute EBV infection. Frequency of intrathoracic lymphadenopathy in setting of acute EBV infection is difficult to illicit given so few patients receive chest X-rays for further diagnostic evaluation [20]. Resolution of hilar and mediastinal lymph adenopathy can take months to resolve [20].

Immunocompromised and pregnant patients are susceptible to developing pneumonia with VZV infection. Radiographic findings include ground glass opacities, consolidation, and uncommon development of bilateral hilar lymphadenopathy [21]. Case reports have also described mediastinal lymphadenopathy in patients with acute influenza infection [22].

Diagnostic Workup

Tuberculosis

Diagnostic workup in tuberculosis is directed at diagnosing and treating patients with active disease and identifying individuals at high risk of latent disease. Most immunocompetent patients will mount an immune cell mediated response that will either clear the initial infection or allow it to remain latent. Treatment of patients with latent disease can reduce risk of reactivation by at much as 90% [24]. Patients with increased risk of new TB infection who warrant screening through tuberculin skin testing (TST) or interferon gamma release assay (IGRA) include individuals with increased risk of tuberculosis exposure and those at increased risk of reactivation due to underlying conditions [23].

Individuals with positive IGRA or TST tests require exclusion of active pulmonary disease as this affects treatment regiment and length. Careful evaluation through history taking, physical examination, and chest imaging can be used to guide further diagnostic testing. Individuals with prolonged cough over 2 weeks with fever, night sweats, and weight loss with an abnormal chest radiograph warrant collection of three sputum specimens [25]. Diagnosis of pulmonary TB can be made from isolation of the organism from bodily secretions or tissue. Sputum samples should be attempted to be collected first and be sent for acid-fast bacilli (AFB) smear, nucleic acid amplification (NAA), and mycobacterial culture.

Sputum may be collected spontaneously or through induction from inhalation of hypertonic saline via nebulizer [26]. Patients unable to produce adequate samples should be considered for bronchoscopy with bronchoalveolar lavage (BAL). Other indications for BAL include individuals with negative sputum samples and high clinical suspicion for TB and those whom alternative diagnose that require bronchoscopy is being considered [27]. When BAL is not diagnostic, transbronchial tissue biopsy may be considered for histopathological examination and microbiology studies. Endobronchial ultrasound with transbronchial needle aspiration (EBUS-TBNA) and endoscopic ultrasound with transesophageal FNA (EUS-FNA) are newer complimentary techniques to further evaluate mediastinal lymphadenopathy. EUS features of TB include predominantly hypoechoic center with preserved or absent borders. Hyperechoic foci can also be seen representing necrotic debris, air, or calcification. A retrospective study confirmed the diagnosis of 61% of cases using EUS-FNA.

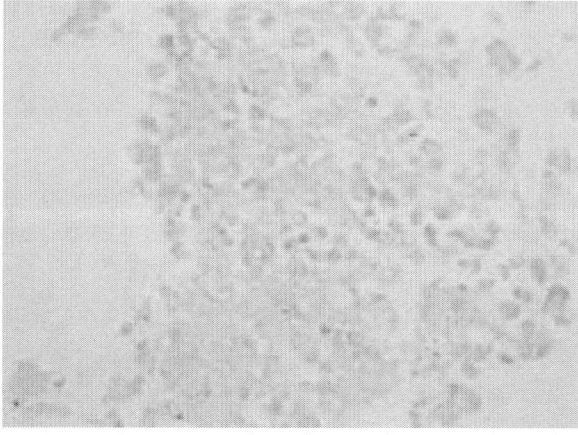

Figure 1. EBUS-TBNA sample showing AFB. Image courtesy Dr. Vikas Pathak.

Individuals with pleural effusion and risk factors for TB contraction should be considered for thoracentesis. Diagnosis of TB pleural effusion can be made with identification or the organism in pleural fluid or pleural biopsy specimens. Thoracentesis should be performed in patients with suspected diagnosis of TB and those who have TB and alternative etiologies of pleural effusion are being considered. Even without histopathological confirmation of TB in pleural fluid, presumptive diagnosis can be made with adenosine deaminase (ADA) levels over 40 units/L and lymphocytic to neutrophil ratio greater than 0.75.

Definitive diagnosis may not be established in 15 to 20% of patients [28]. Empiric therapy should be provided in context of history, radiographic findings, TST/IGRA results, and histopathological results.

Histoplasmosis

Histoplasmosis should be considered in the appropriate epidemiological setting in individuals with hilar and mediastinal masses or lymphadenopathy, pulmonary nodules, or cavitary pulmonary disease. Antigen detection, microscopy and histopathology, culture, and serology can be used for diagnosis. Sensitivity for laboratory-based studies varies based on clinical severity of the illness. The choice of each test used should be applied to the individual's clinical presentation and host factors. For example, serology is the most sensitive laboratory test for detection of self-limited, acute or subacute, and chronic disease, however antigen detection is the most sensitive test for disseminated infection.

Histological examination through bone marrow biopsy or aspirate, BAL sampling, or tissue sampling can be analyzed for diagnosis. Peripheral blood smear can show intracellular organisms in patients with disseminated disease. Of these techniques bone marrow biopsy may be the most rapid method of establishing diagnosis. Sputum cultures may be collected spontaneously, through induction, or BAL. Cultures yield low sensitivity and may take weeks to grow the fungus making it an impractical in the diagnosis of an acutely ill patient.

Various serological markers for antibody detection have been studied including immunodiffusion, complement fixation, latex agglutination, and ELISA. Of these methods immunodiffusion and complement fixation are the two most commonly used modalities due to their accuracy, convenience, and availability. Immunodiffusion has 70 to 100% sensitivity and 100% specificity with diagnosis. Complement fixation with yeast phase antigen has sensitivity of 95% and specificity of 70 to 80%. Drawbacks of these serological tests include delayed onset of development of antibodies after initial histoplasmosis infection resulting in reduced sensitivity and cross reactivity with other fungal pathogens resulting in decreased specificity.

Antigen testing is useful in the acute setting, especially in severely immunocompromised individuals who may not develop adequate antibody response. Sensitivity and specificity in disseminated disease is 95% and 96% respectively however drops to 48% and 96% in non-disseminated disease due to low fungal burden and failure to detect antigens in the serum.

Coccidiodomycosis

Coccidioidomycoses infection is primarily evaluated through serological testing. Most individuals with acute infection will develop symptoms within one to three weeks of inoculation. Antibodies are developed over this time and can be detected through the use of enzyme-linked immunoassays (EIA) and immunodiffusion. EIA testing for serum IgM and IgG are considered first line tests with high sensitivity (83%) for detection of early infection. Immunodiffusion is done to further support the diagnosis given the test's low sensitivity (60.2%) and high specificity (98.8%). These tests are limited in their ability to detect antibodies during the acute stages of infection. If coccidiodoymycosis infection is suspected, weekly EIA testing should be performed as antibodies may develop weeks after acute infection, especially in immunocompromised individuals.

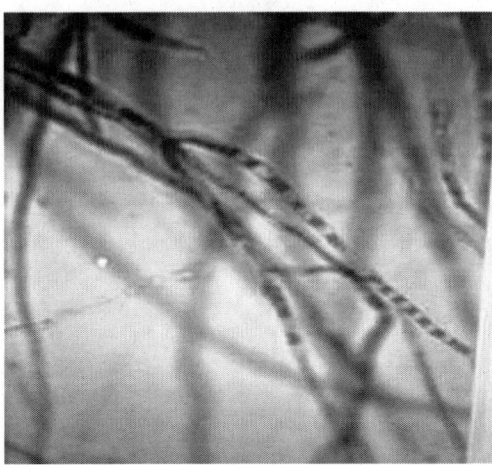

Figure 2. BAL sample showing growth of coccidioidomycosis. Image courtesy, Dr. Vikas Pathak.

Positive immunodiffusion and EIA testing warrant further testing with complement fixation or quantative immunodiffusion. Titers from these tests can be used to monitor treatment response. Coccidiodal antigen is useful in immunocompromised individuals who fail to mount an appropriate immunological response. Testing can be performed on blood and urine, and on cerebrospinal fluid of patients with suspected coccidiodal meningitis. C. Immitis DNA can be amplified using polymerase chain reaction. Use of real time PCR has shown to yield sensitivity of 100% and specificity of 98% when compared to culture [29]. When PCR is used as standard test sensitivity dropped to 56% compared to 44% for fungal culture [30].

Definitive diagnosis can be made by identification of the fungus in blood, tissue samples, sputum, and other body fluid. In tissue samples, a mature spherule of C. immitis with endospores is pathogamonic of infection. Purulent sputum cultures can also establish diagnosis with colonies growing as soon as three to four days. If pulmonary infection is suspected and sputum cannot be obtained spontaneously or through induction, BAL and fine needle aspiration may be needed. Lung biopsy through endoscopic ultrasound or bronchoscopy may be required in immunocompromised individuals with negative sputum and BAL cultures. It is important that laboratory personnel are notified of suspected coccidiodal infection, as mature cultures are very contagious and should be handled with appropriate safety equipment.

Viral Infection

Various viral etiologies are implicated in bilateral hilar and mediastinal lymphadenopathy. Diagnosis of viral infections can be made by culture, serology, EIA, PCR, and immunofluorescence techniques. Diagnostic approaches vary based on the suspected pathogen. For EBV a heterophile antibody test can detect EBV with 85% sensitivity and 100% specificity. A negative test with high clinical suspicion can be evaluated further with EBV antibodies with a sensitivity of 97% and specificity of 94%. PCR can detect EBV DNA with 90% accuracy two weeks after symptoms onset. VZV can be diagnosed using PCR with 95% sensitivity. Diagnosis of VZV and measles virus infection can be made with high sensitivity and specificity using reverse transcriptase PCR.

TREATMENT STRATEGIES

Tuberculosis

Latent and active pulmonary TB differs in their treatment regiments and duration. Latent TB can be treated with one of four regiments. Regiments are highlighted in table one and include the following: Isoniazid (INH) alone for 6 to 9 months, rifampin alone for 4 months, rifampin plus isoniazid for 3 months, rifapentine and isoniazid for 3 months. INH alone has been found to reduce incidence of active pulmonary TB by 60 to 90% in clinical trials. Studies comparing rifampin alone and INH found better compliance, less toxicity, and no inferiority in prevention of active TB with rifampin alone. INH and rifampin combined compared to INH alone found equal efficacy and toxicity rates.

The standard approach to active pulmonary TB involves treatment with rifampin, ethambutol, pyrazinamide, and isoniazid for a 2-month induction phase followed by 4 consolidation phases consisting of isoniazid and rifampin. After two months of initial therapy most patients no longer have viable mycobacteria in their sputum, however an additional 4 months must be completed to avoid relapse. Six month regimens are found to have higher compliance rates and similar rates of relapse (3.5%) compared to longer treatment regiments. Relapse rates can be attributed to noncompliance, drug resistance and poor drug penetration of sequestered mycobacteria. Clinical monitoring is assessed with monthly AFB smear and cultures until two consecutive cultures are negative. A chest radiograph is collected at the end of therapy to use as a baseline.

Mono drug resistant TB is defined as TB resistant to isoniazid. The preferred regiment for treatment is rifampin, pyrazinamide, levofloxacin, and ethambutol [31]. Multidrug resistant (MDR) TB is defined as TB resistant to both isoniazid and rifampin. Therapy for MDR TB is an individualized and prolonged course depending on patient preference, comorbidities, and pregnancy status. The longer individualized oral regiment consists of an intensive phase of respiratory floroquinolones, bedaquiline, linezolid and clofazimine or either cycloserine and terizidone given for six months following sputum culture seroconversion. The continuation phase consists of giving the aforementioned regiment (except for bedaquiline or other injectable) for an additional 15 to 17 months beyond sputum seroconversion. A short-standardized regimen consists of an induction phase of four months with 7 drugs followed by a continuation phase of five months with four drugs. The World Health Organization highlights specific regiments for individuals with various forms of MDR TB.

Histoplasmosis

Mild to moderate histoplasmosis with symptoms less than 4 weeks in duration does not require treatment with antifungals. For those with prolonged symptoms over 4 weeks, itraconazole can be given for a total of

12 weeks. Severe disease with hypoxia and dyspnea concerning for acute respiratory distress syndrome should be treated with amphotericin for one to two weeks followed by a 12-week course of itraconazole. Chronic cavitary histoplasmosis should be treated with a one-year course of intraconazole with some experts suggesting a prolonged 18 to 24-month course for relapse prevention.

Coccidiodomycosis

Immunocompetent patients without evidence of extensive infection or risk factors for infectious progression do not require antifungal therapy. Nonpregnant patients can be treated with a three to six-month course of itraconazole or fluconazole. Amphotericin B is reserved for those with severely extensive disease and immunocompromised states.

Viral Infection

Effective antiviral therapy is not available for most respiratory viruses with treatment focused on symptomatic management. Acute influenza pneumonia can be treated with rapid initiation of oseltamivir. VZV can be treated with acyclovir.

REFERENCES

[1] Ferrer R., Lymphadenopathy: differential diagnosis and evaluation, *Am. Fam. Physician* 58 (1998) 1313-1320.

[2] Schwartza, L. H., Bogaertsb, J., R. Fordc, L. Shankard, P. Therassee, S. Gwytherf, et al., Evaluation of lymph nodes with RECIST 1.1, *Eur. J. Cancer* 45 (2009) 261-267.

[3] Glazer, G. M., Gross, B. H., Quint, L. E., Francis, I. R., Bookstein, F. L., Orringer, M. B. Normal mediastinal lymph nodes: number and size

according to American Thoracic Society mapping. *AJR Am J Roentgenol* 1985;144: 261–265.

[4] Suwatanapongched, T., Gierada, D. S., CT of thoracic lymph nodes. Part II: dis- eases and pitfalls, *Br. J. Radiol.* 79 (2006) 999-1000.

[5] Bayanati, H., Tornhill, E., Souza, C. A., Sethi-Virmani, V., Gupta, A., Maziak, D., et al., Quantitative CT texture and shape analysis: can it differentiate benign and malignant mediastinal lymph nodes in patients with primary lung cancer? *Eur. Radiol.* 25 (2015) 480-487.

[6] Ganeshalingam, S., Koh, D. M., Nodal staging, *Cancer Imaging* 9 (2009) 104-111.

[7] Braun, Carie Ann; Anderson, Cindy Miller (2007). *Pathophysiology: Functional Alterations in Human Health.* Lippincott Williams & Wilkins. p. 326.

[8] Kumar, Vinay; Abbas, Abul K.; Fausto, Nelson; & Mitchell, Richard N. (2007). *Robbins Basic Pathology* (8th ed.). Saunders Elsevier. pp. 516-522.

[9] Burrill, J., Williams, C. J., Bain, G., Conder, G., Hine, A. L., Misra, R. R., Tuberculosis: a radiologic review, *Radiographics* 27 (2007) 1255-1257.

[10] Woodring, J. H., Vandiviere, H. M., Fried, A. M., Dillon, M. L., Williams, T. D., Melvin, I. G. Update: the radio- graphic features of pulmonary tuberculosis. *AJR* 1986; 146:497–506.

[11] Im, J. G., Itoh, H., Shim, Y. S., et al. Pulmonary tuber- culosis: CT findings—early active disease and sequential change with antituber- culous therapy. *Radiology* 1993; 186:653–660.

[12] Chu JH, Feudtner C, Heyden K, Walsh TJ, Zaoutis TE. (2006). Hospitalization for endemic mycosis: a population–based national study. *Clin Infect Dis*, 42, 822–5.

[13] R. Kurowski, M. Ostapchuk, Overview of histoplasmosis, *Am. Fam. Physician* 66 (2002) 2247-2252.

[14] Fojtasek, M. F., Sherman, M. R., Garringer, T., Blair, R., Wheat, L. J., and Schmzlein-Bictc, C. T. (1993). Local immunity in lung-associated lymph nodes in a murine model of pulmonary histoplasmosis. *Infect. Immun.* 61, 4607.

[15] Goodwin, R. A., Loyd, J. E., Des Prez, R. M. Histoplasmosis in normal hosts. *Medicine* (Baltimore) 1981; 60:231–66.

[16] Loyd, J. E., Tillman, B. F., Atkinson, J. B., des Prez, R. M., Mediastinal fibrosis complicating histoplasmosis, *Med. Baltim.* 67 (1988) 295-310.

[17] Goodwin, R. A., Jr., F. T. Owens, J. D. Snell, W. W. Hubbard, R. D. Buchanan, R. T. Terry, and R. M. des Prez. 1976. Chronic pulmonary histoplasmosis. *Medicine* (Baltimore) 55:413–452.

[18] Capone, D., Marchiori, E., Wanke, B., Dantas, K. E., Cavalcanti, M. A., Deus-Filho, A., et al., Acute pulmonary coccidioidomycosis: CT findings from 15 patients, *Br. J. Radiol.* 81 (2008) 721-724.

[19] Thompson, G. R., Pulmonary coccidioidomycosis, *Semin. Respir. Crit. Care. Med.* 32 (2011) 754-763.

[20] Friedland, J. S., Santis, G., Smith, M. J., Infectious mononucleosis: a cause of bilateral hilar lymphadenopathy, *Postgrad. Med. J.* 64 (1988) 799-800.

[21] Maher, T. M., Gupta, N. K., Burke, M. M., Carby, M. R., CT findings of varicella pneumonia after lung transplantation, *AJR Am. J. Roentgenol.* 188 (2007) W557-W559.

[22] VerrastroI, C. G. Y., Abreu-Junior, L., HitomiI, D. Z., AntonioI, E. P., Neves, R. A., D'Ippolito, G., Manifestations of infection by the novel influenza A (H1N1) virus at chest computed tomography, *Radiol. Bras.* 42 (2009) 343-348.

[23] K. Bibbins-Domingo, D. C. Grossman, S. J. Curry, L. Bauman, K. W. Davidson, J. W. Epling Jr., et al. Screening for latent tuberculosis infection in adults: US Preventive Services Task Force recommendation statement *JAMA*, 316 (2016), pp. 962-969.

[24] Comstock, G. W. How much isoniazid is needed for prevention of tuberculosis among immunocompetent adults? *Int J Tuberc Lung Dis* 1999; 3:847-50.

[25] Day, J. H., Charalambous, S., Fielding, K. L., Hayes, R. J., Churchyard, G. J., Grant, A. D. Screening for tuberculosis prior to isoniazid preventive therapy among HIV-infected gold miners in South Africa. *Int J Tuberc Lung Dis* 2006; 10:523–9.

[26] Schoch O, Rieder P, Tueller C, Altpeter E, Zellweger J, Rieder H, Krause M, Thurnheer R. Diagnostic yield of sputum, induced sputum, and bronchoscopy after radiologic tuberculosis screening. *Am J Respir Crit Care Med* 2007; 175:80.

[27] Somu N, Swaminathan S, Paramasivan CN, et al. Value of bronchoalveolar lavage and gastric lavage in the diagnosis of pulmonary tuberculosis in children. *Tuber Lung Dis* 1995;76: 295–9.

[28] Taylor Z, Marks SM, Rios Burrows NM, Weis SE, Stricof RL, Miller B. Causes and costs of hospitalization of tuberculosis patients in the United States. *Int J Tuberc Lung Dis* 2000;4: 931–939.

[29] Binnicker MJ, Buckwalter SP, Eisberner JJ, Stewart RA, McCullough AE, Wohlfiel SL, Wengenack NL. Detection of *Coccidioides* species in clinical specimens by real-time PCR. *J Clin Microbiol.* 2007;45: 173–8.

[30] Kerrick SS, Lundergan LL, Galgiani JN. Coccidioidomycosis at a university health service. *Am Rev Respir Dis* 1985;131: 100–102.

[31] Menzies D, Benedetti A, Paydar A, et al. Standardized treatment of active tuberculosis in patients with previous treatment and/or with mono-resistance to isoniazid: a systematic review and meta-analysis. *PLoS Med* 2009;6: 1000150-1000150.

In: Thoracic Lymphadenopathy
Editor: Vikas Pathak

ISBN: 978-1-53616-700-9
© 2020 Nova Science Publishers, Inc.

Chapter 6

SARCOIDOSIS

Christina Mutch, DO and Vikas Pathak, MD
Riverside Regional Medical Center,
Newport News, Virginia, US

EPIDEMIOLOGY

First described as a separate entity in the late 19th century by a Scandinavian dermatologist, sarcoidosis was first thought to be an isolated skin disease. Now, more than 150 years later, we know that is far from the case. Although sarcoidosis affects ethnicities worldwide, there are significant differences in both prevalence and severity among these groups. Overall, African-Americans and Nordic populations have the highest incidence and prevalence [1]. In the US, African Americans not only have a higher prevalence (approximately 36 in 100,000 vs 10.9 in 100,000 in American Caucasians) they also have a 7.5 times higher risk of hospitalization and mortality [2].

In terms of age distribution, approximately 68% of those with the disease are less than 40 years old. In African American women, it is more commonly in the 4th decade of life. Recent studies are suggesting that there may be a bimodal distribution with incidence occurring around 20-40 and then after age 55 [3].

PATHOPHYSIOLOGY

The exact mechanisms and causes of sarcoidosis are not entirely understood, and it is ultimately still classified as an unknown mechanism under the broader umbrella of non-caseating granulomatous interstitial lung diseases. The leading theory for sarcoidosis is an environmental trigger(s) incites a local inflammatory response, leading to activation of TH1 CD4 immune cells, which in turn, secrete inflammatory factors such as Interleukin-2 and IFN-gamma leading to further recruitment of additional Th1 cells and macrophages. Ultimately, the cascade of effects results in epithelioid cell granuloma formation and in some cases, fibrosis. Approximately 20-25% of patients go on to develop pulmonary fibrosis [4]. The hunt for genetic and environmental causes that trigger this cascade continues. Although a wide array of environmental antigens and genes have been implicated, currently, the two leading targets are HLA-DQB1 and HLA-DRB1 and exposure to water damage or high humidity in the workplace [4]. Although microbes have been studied as possible inciting causes, no definitive data exists for any one microbe.

CLINICAL CHARACTERISTICS

With greater than 87% of patients having pulmonary involvement, it is not surprising that the most common presentation involves respiratory symptoms of dyspnea on exertion, shortness of breath and dry cough. Patients can also experience night sweats, fatigue and weight loss. Common skin manifestations include erythema nodosum (which will not have the classic histopathology of sarcoidosis) and violaceous papules of lupus pernio. Eye involvement includes uveitis, episcleritis, clogged tear ducts, increase in intraocular pressure and even blindness. Nervous system involvement manifests most commonly with CN VII or Bell's Palsy, but can occur nearly anywhere in the CNS or PNS. Still, approximately 50% of cases are asymptomatic, detected by incidental findings on chest radiography [1].

Clinical course varies among patients as much as symptoms. Early stage disease at the time of diagnosis is associated with a better prognosis, with the converse, having stage 2-3 at time of diagnosis, associated with high mortality rates. Other poor prognostic factors include being diagnosed after age 40, black race, hypercalcemia, splenomegaly, osseous involvement, chronic uveitis and lupus pernio. Lofgren Syndrome, which consists of fever, polyarthritis, erythema nodosum, and bilateral lymphadenopathy, is a good prognostic factor often having a spontaneous remission rate of >85% [1].

LABORATORY

Sarcoidosis can classically lead to hypercalcemia but actually only occurs in 11% of patients, while hypercalciuria occurs in approximately 20% [1]. The mechanism for this is due to an increase in conversion of 25OH Vitamin D to activated 1,25 vitamin D by the recruited macrophages that secrete 25-hydroxyvitamin D-1alphahydroxlase [1]. All patients diagnosed with sarcoidosis should undergo a 24-hour urinary excretion of calcium for this reason in addition to serum calcium. Renal failure in sarcoidosis is due to extensive calcium deposition. Granulomatous nephritis is very rare. ACE levels are elevated in approximately 75% of cases, but it is neither sensitive nor specific for the disease, and thus has limited utility [5]. ACE levels can be elevated in a whole host of diseases ranging from hyperthyroidism to lung cancer.

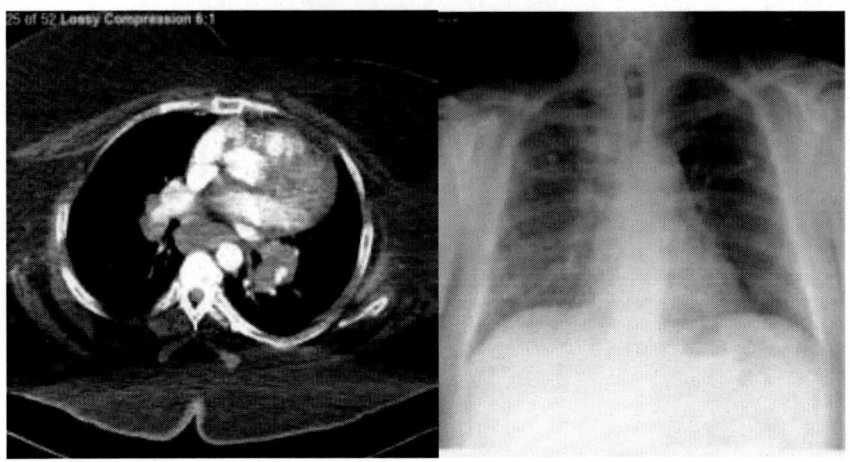

Figure 1. CT chest showing bilateral hilar and mediastinal lymphadenopathy; Chest x-ray showing mediastinal lymphadenopathy.

IMAGING

Imaging plays a pivotal role in aiding in the diagnosis of sarcoidosis. Often, sarcoidosis is first picked up on chest radiographic, with the classic bilateral hilar lymphadenopathy, found in 50-80% of cases [6]. The most common pattern of LAD is bilateral hilar and right paratracheal, known as Garland's triad [7]. The Siltzbach classification system helps estimate prognosis based on chest radiography staging (Table 1). Stage 0 has no radiographic abnormalities. Stage 1 has hilar lymphadenopathy, and 80% of these patients will improve or reach remission. Stage 2, in addition to hilar LAD, also has parenchymal infiltrates, with a 68% chance of improvement. Stage 3 has all the characteristics of Stage 2, but severity of infiltrates is so severe the hilar LAD becomes obscured. Patients with Stage 3 have a 37% chance of improvement [8]. Stage 4 is the most severe and shows signs of fibrocystic changes. It is important to keep in mind that radiographic staging does not correlate with pulmonary function testing.

Abnormal chest radiography often prompts further imaging with High-Resolution CT (HRCT) Thorax. Typical features found on CT include the bilateral hilar lymphadenopathy (95%) [8], peri-lymphangitic spread resulting in a bronchovascular distribution of granulomas found in 75-90% of cases [8]. Also typical is peribronchovascular nodularity, patchy ground-glass opacities (40%). If nodules are seen on CT they are typically multiple, ill-defined, bilateral and usually perihilar and on the periphery. Prevascular nodes, middle mediastinal, left paratracheal, subcarinal or both are present in about 50% of patients. Fibrotic changes can also be seen such as traction bronchiectasis, reticular opacities and volume loss. The upper lung fields are disproportionately affected. This distribution and the fact that distal bronchi are rarely involved, lead to often normal lung sounds on auscultation of the lungs.

No staging system has yet been developed for high-resolution CT. Despite this, HRCT has its own advantages and utility. HRCT has the capability of distinguishing between chronic and acute inflammation and can help clinicians decided on the need for acute treatment. Signs of reversible, acute inflammation on CT include ground-glass opacities, nodules and alveolar opacities. Irreversible, chronic changes present on CT as volume loss (typically in upper lobes), traction bronchiectasis, honeycombing, emphysema, bullae and mycetoma. Calcifications can also be seen in chronic cases, occurring in 20% of patients after 10 years.

Table 1. Sarcoidosis staging based on chest radiography findings.

Stage	CXR Findings	Percentage of Pt w Stage at diagnosis	Chance of Spontaneous Remission
0	No abnormalities	5-10%	
1	Lymphadenopathy (LAD) Only	50%	60-90%
2	LAD + Pulmonary Infiltrates	25-30%	40-70%
3	Pulmonary infiltrates obscuring LAD	10-12%	10-20%
4	Fibrosis	5%	0%

DIFFERENTIAL DIAGNOSIS OF MEDIASTINAL LAD

Although classic clinical and radiographic findings can sometimes be enough to determine the diagnosis of sarcoidosis, atypical features, necessitates the need for further confirmation and a broader differential.

Atypical features include asymmetric, unilateral hilar lymph node enlargement (<5% of sarcoidosis patients), and even more rare, mediastinal lymph nodes without hilar lymph nodes. Pulmonary nodules, masses and airspace consolidation can be seen in around 15%, but again, are not pathognomonic and warrant further delineation.

Typical LAD (bilateral and symmetrical hilar and right paratracheal), can also be seen in malignancies, especially lymphoma, as well as infections. Though, without symptoms, sarcoidosis is the most common diagnosis. Studies have been conducted which aim to determine if imaging alone can predict the risk of lymphoma vs sarcoidosis.

Differential diagnosis for mediastinal lymphadenopathy includes malignancy (metastasis as well as lymphoma), hypersensitivity pneumonitis, and autoimmune pathology such as rheumatoid arthritis, infectious causes, granulomatous disease (in addition to sarcoidosis, berylliosis, granulomatosis with polyangiitis), COPD, CHF, and even Iatrogenic from medications. Commonly used medications include anti-hypertensives such as captopril, atenolol, and hydralazine, as well as antibiotics such as the tetracyclines, isoniazid, cephalosporins, and penicillin, even aspirin, ibuprofen, methotrexate and allopurinol [9-12].

If infection is suspected, bronchial-alveolar lavage (BAL) can play a role to rule out bacterial or fungal causes via respiratory culture. Tuberculosis, histoplasmosis, and coccidioidomycosis are the most common infectious causes that lead to mediastinal lymphadenopathy [12].

To make matters even more complicated, there is a 5.5-11.5 times higher incidence of lymphoma in sarcoidosis patients, Hodgkin's being the more common type. Furthermore, although uncommon to have bilateral lymphadenopathy in lymphoma, silicosis, amyloidosis, or berylliosis, they can commonly have high-density, bilateral LAD and calcifications as seen in sarcoidosis [13].

With the differential being so broad, and the severe implications of missing a cancerous diagnosis, role for other diagnostic modalities have been investigated. FDG-PET/CT was studied as a non-invasive option, in hopes that it would help distinguish between lymphoma and sarcoidosis in lymphadenopathy. When PET was performed in 36 biopsy proven sarcoidosis patients, 78% were picked up on PET scan [3]. There was also a lack of specificity, as PET is about 100% sensitive in lung cancer. Additionally, PET/CT could not distinguish between sarcoidosis and sarcoid reaction [3]. Thus, invasive techniques for biopsy remains pivotal.

Diagnosis

Typically, a definitive diagnosis is obtained via direct biopsy of an involved organ, preferably the least invasive target. In addition to histopathology, sarcoid-like reaction, which as similar biopsy findings, must be ruled out. Sarcoid-like reaction is granuloma formation in reaction to *known* conditions, including, but not limited to: fungal diseases, tuberculosis, berylliosis, leprosy, Crohn's disease, primary biliary cirrhosis [2]. Several modes for biopsy can be used, depending on the location of lymph node, including CT-guided, blind transbronchial needle aspiration (TBNA) or surgical. TBNA can be used for large (>1.5 cm) lymph nodes, limited to mediastinal area, including right paratracheal, subcarinal, and hilum areas. Sensitivity for TBNA for lung cancer is only 40% [8].

A recent advancement, Endobronchial ultrasonography (EBUS), provides a minimally invasive way of obtaining biopsy through fine needle-aspiration under direct visualization. It has a sensitivity for lung cancer of 90% including in lymph nodes <1.5 cm [8]. Additionally, EBUS can access more sites and give direct visualized for macroscopic characterization of the lymph node. Naturally, EBUS was studied in use for sarcoidosis, and studies confirmed higher sensitivity and specificity compared to blind TBNA [1, 9, 10].

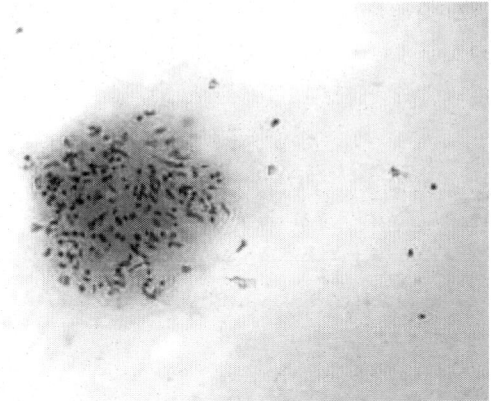

Figure 2. EBUS-TBNA sample obtained from lymph node shows granuloma.

HISTOPATHOLOGY

Once biopsy is obtained, pathology demonstrates the classic non-caseous granulomas, with fibroblasts and collagen present in the surrounding tissue. The center of the granulomas contains multinucleated giant cells, lymphocytes and epithelioid cells. Central necrosis is not typical. Overtime, the granulomas can become surrounded by fibrous tissue or even completely replaced by hyaline fibrous scars [7].

TREATMENT

Many cases do not requirement treatment, and 2/3 of cases spontaneously go into remission [6]. For more severe cases, treatment is chosen based on the involved organ and most typically involve some sort of glucocorticoid therapy (with organ dependent dosing and route). For involved skin issues, other anti-inflammatories can be used, such as hydroxychloroquine, methotrexate or even thalidomide. Treatment for lung disease is guided by regular PFTs. Approximately 3% of lung transplants go to sarcoidosis patients, and the survival rates post-transplant are similar to the general lung transplant population [6].

REFERENCES

[1] Koo, Hyun Jung, & Choi, Chang-Min, et al. (2015). Evaluation of Mediastinal Lymph Nodes in Sarcoidosis, Sarcoid Reaction, and Malignant Lymph Nodes Using CT and FDG-PET/CT. *Medicine,* 94(27):1-9.

[2] Gerke, Alicia, & Koth, Laura, et al. (2017). Disease Burden and Variability in Sarcoidosis. *Annals of American Thoracic Society*, 17(6): S421-S428.

[3] Criado, Eva & Exaubet, Antonio, et al. (2010). Pulmonary Sarcoidosis: Typical and Atypical Manifestations at High-Resolution CT with pathologic Correlation. *Radiographics*, 30:1567-1586.

[4] Iannuzzi, Michael & Teirstein, Alvin, et al. (2017). Sarcoidosis. *New England Journal of Medicine,* 357: 2153-2165.

[5] Arkema, Elizabeth, et al. Epidemiology of Sarcoidosis: Current Findings and Future Directions. (2018). *Therapeutic Advances in Chronic Disease,* 9(11) 227-240.

[6] Nunes, Hilario, et al. (2012). Imaging of sarcoidosis of the airways and lung parenchyma and correlation with lung function. *European Respiratory Journal,* 40(3): 750-765.

[7] Robbins, et al. (2010) *Pathologic Basis of Disease*. 8th edition. Saunders Elsevier. 701-702.

[8] Silvestri, G. A. (2009). The mounting evidence for endobronchial ultrasound. *Chest,* 136(2)327-328.

[9] Tremblay, A., Stather, D. R., MacEachern, P, et al. (2009). A randomized controlled trial of standard versus endobronchial ultrasound guided transbronchial needle aspiration in patients with suspected sarcoidosis. *Chest*, 136:340-346.

[10] Garwood, S., et al. (2007). Endobronchial ultrasound for the diagnosis of pulmonary sarcoidosis. *Chest*, 132(4): 1298-1304.

[11] Ungprasert, P., Carmona, E. M, Crowson, C. S., Matteson, E. L, et al. (2016) Diagnostic Utility of Angiotensin Converting Enzyme in Sarcoidosis: A Population-Based Study. *Lung,* 194(1):91-95.

[12] Nin, Carlos Schuler, et al. (2016). Thoracic lymphadenopathy in benign diseases: A state of the art review. *Respiratory Medicine*. 112:10-17.

Chapter 7

INTERSTITIAL AND OCCUPATIONAL LUNG DISEASES

Darrin Hursey[1], MD, Michael Shallcross[2] and Vikas Pathak[2], MD

[1]WakeMed Health and Hospitals, Raleigh, North Carolina, US
[2]Riverside Regional Medical Center, Newport News, Virginia, US

INTERSTITIAL LUNG DISEASES

Introduction

Mediastinal lymphadenopathy is typically defined as an increase in size of the mediastinal lymph nodes to greater than 1cm in short axis on chest CT. The thoracic lymph nodes are divided into 14 separate locations, or stations, based upon classic surgical landmarks. This allows for a standardized description of lymph node location and consistent nomenclature across varied disciplines. Stations 1-9 represent nodes that are more central, while the nodes in stations 10-14 are more peripheral [1]. This distinction is most pertinent with regards to lung cancer, as it is a critical component of the staging process.

Hilar and mediastinal lymphadenopathy is seen in a diverse array of diseases. Various malignancies, including lymphoma and advanced lung, breast, or upper GI cancer can present with mediastinal lymphadenopathy. A wide variety of benign conditions can also manifest this feature. Infectious causes include tuberculosis and the endemic mycoses such as histoplasmosis or coccidioidomycosis. Other conditions featuring hilar and mediastinal lymphadenopathy include sarcoidosis, congestive heart failure, chronic obstructive pulmonary disease, and interstitial lung disease [2] [table 1]. As part of the discussion of mediastinal lymphadenopathy in interstitial lung disease, a brief overview of these disorders follows.

Interstitial lung disease is a term that describes a very heterogeneous group of disorders that share the common feature of diffuse involvement of the lung parenchyma, beginning in the interstitium. In the broadest terms, the interstitial lung diseases are divided into the disorders of known cause and those of unknown etiology. Examples of the former include drug or radiation effects, environmental exposures, and connective tissue disease. The latter group includes sarcoidosis and the idiopathic interstitial pneumonias [3].

The idiopathic interstitial pneumonias are further divided into the rare, major, and unclassifiable idiopathic pneumonias. The major idiopathic interstitial pneumonias include the most commonly encountered disorders, such as idiopathic pulmonary fibrosis, nonspecific interstitial pneumonia, cryptogenic organizing pneumonia (previously known as BOOP), and acute interstitial pneumonia [4] (Table 2).

Arguably, the most important distinction amongst the idiopathic interstitial pneumonias is that between Idiopathic Pulmonary Fibrosis and the rest. Idiopathic Pulmonary Fibrosis has a very distinctive appearance with regards to its underlying histology, clinical presentation and natural history, and radiographic appearance [5]. In fact, its radiographic appearance is often sufficiently specific as to allow confident diagnosis without the benefit of biopsy confirmation.

The critical component of the evaluation of interstitial lung disease is the chest CT. Computed tomography provides an evaluation of the lung parenchyma and other thoracic structures that is far superior to older modalities. Chest CT can demonstrate reticular infiltrates, traction bronchiectasis, ground glass opacities, and honeycomb changes (clusters of cysts that are typically subpleural) that are difficult or impossible to discern on standard chest radiography [5]. The presence of these findings and their distribution in the lung fields can help suggest the identity of the underlying disorder. While scoring systems exist that utilize these chest CT findings to predict survival in interstitial lung disease [6], they tend to be difficult to apply in clinical practice for a number of reasons [7].

One finding that is readily apparent on chest CT in interstitial lung disease, but has perhaps been underappreciated, is lymphadenopathy. Hilar and mediastinal lymphadenopathy is increasingly recognized as a common, potentially clinically significant feature in these diseases. The precise pathophysiology to explain the development of lymphadenopathy in interstitial lung disease in unclear, but it is felt to be likely due to an inflammatory response that ultimately results in lymphoid hyperplasia [8, 9].

Studies in the late 20th century reported an increased prevalence of hilar and mediastinal lymphadenopathy in patients with interstitial lung disease. Mediastinal adenopathy was seen in over 60% of patients with idiopathic pulmonary fibrosis and over 80% of those with sarcoidosis [10, 11]. There were relatively few patients with other forms of interstitial lung disease in these fairly small studies, and no clinical significance was sought regarding the presence of lymphadenopathy in these patients.

This question of clinical significance was investigated in subsequent studies. A small study in 2000 demonstrated a correlation between the number of lymph nodes and their size with CT severity scores [8]. A later study examined a wider variety of interstitial lung diseases and again found a high prevalence of hilar and mediastinal lymphadenopathy in these conditions. No correlation was found between lymph node characteristics and any particular subtype of interstitial lung disease, so it was concluded that lymphadenopathy was not useful in differentiating between these various diseases [9].

More recently, a much larger study which included over 1000 patients with a wide variety of interstitial lung disease suggested that the presence of mediastinal lymphadenopathy in these patients was clinically relevant in a number of ways. The presence of enlarged mediastinal lymph nodes was associated with a significantly lower rate of transplant free survival, significantly lower lung function, and significantly increased rate of hospitalization for respiratory complications [12]. Mortality increased with both increasing number and size of mediastinal lymph nodes, even when adjusting for other relevant variables. These findings occurred across interstitial lung disease subtypes.

This suggests that prognostic information can be gleaned from not just the parenchymal findings on chest CT, but also from the evaluation of the hilar and mediastinal lymph nodes that these examinations provide. As has been noted previously, utilizing the parenchymal characteristics for prognostic purposes in these patients is challenging. The number and size of hilar and mediastinal lymph nodes could be a more practical and useful marker for disease severity; this could help guide monitoring and treatment decisions. Treatment of interstitial lung disease can pose many challenges, including cost and a high side effect burden. This is particularly true in Idiopathic Pulmonary Fibrosis. Newly developed treatments are very expensive and can often have intolerable side effects [13], so determining which patients should consider these treatments and when is paramount.

In summary, hilar and mediastinal lymphadenopathy is a feature of interstitial lung disease that has not been well appreciated. While the presence of lymphadenopathy on chest CT does not appear to assist in the diagnosis of interstitial lung disease or differentiate between the various subtypes, it does appear to provide prognostic information that can be utilized to guide monitoring and treatment decisions.

Table 1. Benign etiologies of mediastinal lymphadenopathy

Tuberculosis
Histoplasmosis
Coccidioidomycosis
Sarcoidosis
Silicosis
Castleman's disease
Drug reactions
Congestive Heart Failure
Interstitial Lung Disease

Table 2. The idiopathic interstitial pneumonias

Rare:
-Idiopathic Lymphoid Interstitial Pneumonia
-Idiopathic Pleuroparenchymal Fibroelastosis
Major:
-Idiopathic Pulmonary Fibrosis
-Idiopathic Nonspecific Interstitial Pneumonia
-Cryptogenic Organizing Pneumonia
-Acute Interstitial Pneumonia
-Respiratory Bronchiolitis-Interstitial Lung Disease
-Desquamative Interstitial Lung Disease
Unclassifiable Idiopathic Interstitial Pneumonias

OCCUPATIONAL LUNG DISEASES

Introduction

Occupational lung diseases are often work-related lung conditions that present as a direct result of a patient's exposure to a particular agent within their place of work via inhalation or ingestion of dust particles or noxious chemicals. Occupational lung diseases include a broad group of diagnoses and etiologies, but this chapter will focus on three specific exposures; Coal Worker's Pneumoconiosis (CWP), Silicosis, and Berylliosis [14-17]. Most of these disorders present as diffuse lung disease, but the implementation of high-resolution computed tomography (HRCT) allows for further differentiation based on characteristic radiographic findings. However, a combination of clinical features and relevant occupation history in conjunction with imaging modalities can play a key role in the diagnosis and treatment of these diseases.

Coal Worker's Pneumoconiosis

Exposure and Etiology

The primary exposure resulting in the development of CWP is inhalation of washed coal. Coal dust is composed of carbon-containing particles, and as expected, individuals that work in coal mines are at high risk of exposure. In addition, coal miners that drill into rock formations are also at risk of inhaling silica-containing dust as well as kaolin and mica. It is important to note that washed coal is almost completely free of silica, however, CWP and Silicosis are often undifferentiated on high-resolution CT imaging and other radiographic modalities. Despite similarities in imaging, CWP and Silicosis have distinct histological features in addition to particle exposure. Inhalation of coal dust is also related to rapid development and progression of chronic obstructive pulmonary disease (COPD), increasing mortality of patients. Symptoms are typically non-specific and include dyspnea, cough, and production of phlegm.

Histological/Pathological Findings

Due to the presence of charcoal in coal-containing dust particles, CWP is sometimes referred to as the "Black Lung Disease." Tissue specimens and biopsies from patients presenting with CWP contain two characteristic and distinctive morphological features. One feature being the formation of coal macules. These coal macules will range from 1-5 mm in size and are characterized by solid anthracotic pigmentation without fibrous tissue intervention. Macules will also contain pigment-laden macrophages surrounding bronchioles in the centrilobular region of the lungs. The second feature being progressive massive fibrosis, indicated by a fibrotic mass with a diameter larger than 1 cm and associated anthracotic pigmentation. These fibrotic masses often show regions of central necrosis within black-pigmented parenchyma.

In complicated cases of CWP, fibrotic masses will present. These masses will consist of a disordered arrangement of collagen fibers, numerous pigment-filled macrophages, as well as free pigment in the centrilobular regions.

Imaging and Radiologic Findings

In its simpler form, CWP typically presents with a radiographic pattern demonstrating small, round nodular opacities. These opacities will occasionally include reticular or reticulonodular opacities as well. Nodules seen on radiographs will measure 1-5 mm in diameter, with less definition at their margins, and more granular appearing in comparison to Silicosis. Calcifications can be found in 10-20% of patients and present as central nodular lesions. CT findings typically include small nodules presenting diffusely in the lung fields. Nodular distribution is perilymphatic, sometimes centrilobular dominant, and often more numerous in the upper lung fields. Calcification within the nodules is identified in 30% of patients on CT. In addition, hilar or mediastinal lymphadenopathy is also seen in 30% of patients on CT.

In its more complicated form, chest radiographs will show large opacities, indicating progressive massive fibrosis in patients. Most of these fibrotic masses will have an irregular border with surrounding paracicatricial emphysema.

Silicosis

Exposure, Etiology and Clinical Presentation

Silicosis is caused by the inhalation of silica (crystalline silicon dioxide) in its fine particle form. Silica typically originates from quartz and occupations involved in mining, quarrying, foundry working, ceramics manufacturing, sandblasting, and tunneling are associated with Silicosis in patients. Crystalline silica is also naturally occurring in rock, sand, concrete, ceramics, bricks, and tiles. Lung injury will typically occur with the inhalation of silica particles that measure 1-2 mm in size reaching the alveoli in the lungs and subsequently ingested by macrophages. Silica particles have a direct cytotoxic effect, resulting in macrophage death and release of inflammatory cytokines. Cytokine release and the inflammatory response results in the proliferation of fibroblasts. Silicosis has a latency period of 10-30 years, but can present in an acute form if workers are exposed to higher quantities of silica dust over a short period of time, leading to clinical presentation in 6-8 months. As discussed with CWP, Silicosis symptoms are typically non-specific and include progressive dyspnea, cough, and production of phlegm.

Histological/Pathological Findings

Macrophage ingestion and subsequent death results in the release of inflammatory cytokines and a localized response to the site of injury leading to fibroblast proliferation. These fibroblasts will form hyalinized nodules composed of concentric layers of collagen. These concentric layers of collagen will form around the entrapped silica particle(s), leading to the development of a fibrous capsule, and demonstrates Silicosis in its simple form. Silicosis enters its complicated form when the crystalline silica enters the periphery of the entrapped nodules and induce additional fibrotic response. This fibrotic response includes the development of new silicotic nodules and overall massive fibrosis in the lung tissue. The development of progressive massive fibrosis becomes more complicated with the involvement of lymph nodes containing silica-containing macrophages that reach the hila and mediastinum.

Imaging and Radiologic Findings

Radiographic findings in its simple presentation demonstrate calcifications that are more diffuse in nature when compared to CWP patients. This is typically described as a pathognomonic eggshell calcification pattern. On HRCT, simple Silicosis findings include multiple small nodules usually 2-5 mm in size, and sometimes up to 10 mm, localized to the upper and posterior bilateral lung regions. These nodules tend to be concentrated in a centrilobular distribution and in its earliest presentation, may be ill-defined as branching centrilobular opacities with irregular fibrosis surrounding the bronchioles. In addition, coalescence of subpleural nodules containing silica lead to the formation of pseudo plaques. Compared to CWP, hilar and mediastinal lymphadenopathy is often more present in Silicosis patients and often present on HRCT. These hilar and mediastinal lymph nodes may also present with calcification and produce an "eggshell" appearance either diffusely or peripherally. In its acute, progressive forms, findings will include numerous ill-defined centrilobular nodules, patchy ground glass opacity, and lung consolidation on HRCT. Superimposed septal thickening termed "crazy-paving" may also develop, and mimic pulmonary alveolar proteinosis. Once again, hilar and mediastinal lymphadenopathy is also common with possible calcification of the lymph nodes.

In its complicated form, Silicosis is associated heavily with progressive massive fibrosis (PMF). This is due to the expansion and convergence of silicotic nodules forming larger, symmetric opacities on CT measuring greater than 1 cm in diameter, localized to the apical and posterior segments of the upper lung lobes. These larger opacities present with irregular margins and are usually not calcified. Segmental areas with pleural thickness and calcification can also develop with onset of PMF in patients with advanced disease. With disease progression, large fibrotic opacities will migrate towards the hila with decreased lung perfusion, and will be surrounded by smaller nodules. Paracicatricial emphysema interspersed between larger fibrotic opacities and the lung pleura will also be seen. On occasion, larger opacities can become centrally necrotic and show cavitation.

Berylliosis

Exposure, Etiology and Clinical Presentation

Berylliosis, technically a pneumoconiosis, differs in that it is a chronic granulomatous hypersensitivity reaction to inhaled beryllium dust, fumes, and salts. The amount of inhaled particulate and duration of exposure does not correlate directly with incidence and severity of the disease. Beryllium use and exposure is typically found in occupations involving nuclear power, aerospace, ceramics, and metal manufacturing, with dentistry also having ties to the chronic diseased state. The hypersensitivity reaction is characterized by accumulation of CD4+ T-cells and macrophages in the lower respiratory tract of patients. The acute presentation of Berylliosis is rare today in industry due to increased industrial control measures, but there is an increased in recognition in patients that have developed sensitization or chronic forms of the disease, occurring in 1-15% of those exposed. Signs and symptoms include dyspnea on exertion, cough, chest pain, fatigue, fever, anorexia, and weight loss, all of which are non-specific. However, skin lesions are the most common finding outside of the chest wall and may be associated with granulomatous hepatitis, hypercalcemia, and renal calculi. Presentation may develop up to 40 years following exposure.

Histological/Pathological Findings

Histopathological findings of chronic Berylliosis are almost identical to that of Sarcoidosis. They include the formation of non-caseating granulomas with a mononuclear cellular infiltrate. In addition, interstitial fibrosis is sometimes present. Granulomas found in Berylliosis are indistinguishable from other pathological granulomatous lesions. However, in its early stages, beryllium sensitivity can be determined using blood samples or bronchoalveolar lavage fluid for detection of lymphocyte transformation and proliferation. Often, pathologic specimens obtained from the mediastinal lymph nodes will contain multiple non-caseating granulomas and sample testing is required to confirm a diagnosis.

Imaging and Radiologic Findings

Plain chest radiographs present with normal findings in up to 46% of patients in the early diseased state. However, disease progression yields chest radiographs showing reticulonodular opacities predominating in the middle and upper lung zones, bilaterally. In more advanced disease states, interstitial fibrosis with honeycombing or mass lesions may present. The presentation of these mass lesions is likely caused by convergence of the granulomatous lesions. In addition, hilar lymphadenopathy is frequently present on radiographs, but not as predominant or as impressive when compared to Sarcoidosis patients.

HRCT findings are similar to those of other granulomatous lung diseases such as Sarcoidosis. Most commonly, patients will have small, parenchymal nodules predominant along bronchovascular bundles or distributed along the interlobular septa. In addition, interlobular septal thickening is also common. Other findings may also include ground-glass opacities, honeycombing, and bronchial wall thickening, with conglomerate masses presenting rarely in only advanced disease patients. In addition, mediastinal and hilar lymphadenopathy is observed in 25-39% of patients, but is overall less common compared to findings in Sarcoidosis patients.

REFERENCES

[1] Walker, C., Chung, J., Abbott, G., Little, B., et al. Mediastinal Lymph Node Staging: From Noninvasive to Surgical. *AJR* 2012; 199: W54-W64.

[2] Nin, C., de Souza, V., Amaral, R., Neto, R., Alves, G., et al. Thoracic lymphadenopathy in benign diseases: A state of the art review. *Respiratory Medicine* 2016; 112: 10-17.

[3] American Thoracic Society, European Respiratory Society. American Thoracic Society/European Respiratory Society international multi-disciplinary consensus classification of the idiopathic interstitial pneumonias. *Am J Respir Crit Care Med* 2002; 165:277–304.

[4] Travis, W. D., Costabel, U., Hansell, D. M., King Jr., T. E., Lynch, D. A., Nicholson, A. G., et al.; ATS/ERS Committee on Idiopathic Interstitial Pneumonias. An official American Thoracic Society/ European Respiratory Society statement: update of the international multidisciplinary classification of the idiopathic interstitial pneumonias. *Am J Respir Crit Care Med* 2013; 188:733–748.

[5] Raghu, G., Collard, H. R., Egan, J. J., Martinez, F. J., Behr, J., Brown, K. K., et al.; ATS/ERS/JRS/ALAT Committee on Idiopathic Pulmonary Fibrosis. An official ATS/ERS/JRS/ALAT statement: idiopathic pulmonary fibrosis: evidence-based guidelines for diagnosis and management. *Am J Respir Crit Care Med* 2011; 183:788–824.

[6] Ryerson, C. J., Vittinghoff, E., Ley, B., Lee, J. S., Mooney, J. J., Jones, K. D., et al. Predicting survival across chronic interstitial lung disease: the ILD-GAP model. *Chest* 2014; 145:723–728.

[7] Walsh, S. Mediastinal lymphadenopathy in Interstitial Lung Disease: Time to be counted. *Am J Respir Crit Care Med* 2019; 199: 685-687.

[8] Jung, J. I., Kim, H. H., Jung, Y. J., Park, S. H., Lee, J. M., Hahn, S. T., Mediastinal lymphadenopathy in pulmonary fibrosis: correlation with disease severity. *J. Comput. Assist. Tomogr* 2000; 24: 706-710.

[9] Souza, C. A., Muller, N. L., Lee, K. S., Johkoh, T. T., Mitsuhiro, H., Chong, S., Idiopathic interstitial pneumonias: prevalence of mediastinal lymph node enlargement in 206 patients. *AJR Am. J. Roentgenol* 2006; 168: 995-999.

[10] Niimi, H., Kang, E. Y., Kwong, J. S., Carignan, S., Müller, N. L., CT of chronic infiltrative lung disease: prevalence of mediastinal lymphadenopathy. *J. Comput. Assist. Tomogr* 2006; 20: 305-308.

[11] Lim, M. K., Im, J. G., Ahn, J. M., Kim, J. H., Lee, S. K., Yeon, K. M., et al., Idiopathic pulmonary fibrosis vs. pulmonary involvement of collagen vascular disease: HRCT findings. *J. Korean Med. Sci* 1997; 12: 492-498.

[12] Adegunsoye, A., Oldham, J. M., Bonham, C., Hrusch, C., Nolan, P., Klejch, W., et al. Prognosticating outcomes in interstitial lung disease by mediastinal lymph node assessment: an observational cohort study

with independent validation. *Am J Respir Crit Care Med* 2019; 199:747–759.

[13] Raghu, G., Rochwerg, B., Zhang, Y., Garcia, C. A., Azuma, A., Behr, J., et al.; American Thoracic Society; European Respiratory society; Japanese Respiratory Society; Latin American Thoracic Association. An official ATS/ERS/JRS/ALAT clinical practice guideline: treatment of idiopathic pulmonary fibrosis. An update of the 2011 clinical practice guideline. *Am J Respir Crit Care Med* 2015;192: e3–e19.

[14] Chong, S., Lee, K. S., Chung, M. J., Han, J., Kwon, O. J., & Kim, T. S. (2006). Pneumoconiosis: comparison of imaging and pathologic findings. *Radiographics*, *26*(1), 59-77.

[15] Kim, K. I., Kim, C. W., Lee, M. K., Lee, K. S., Park, C. K., Choi, S. J., & Kim, J. G. (2001). Imaging of occupational lung disease. *Radiographics*, *21*(6), 1371-1391.

[16] Meyer, K. C. (1994). Beryllium and lung disease. *Chest*, *106*(3), 942-946.

[17] Sirajuddin, A., & Kanne, J. P. (2009). Occupational lung disease. *Journal of thoracic imaging*, *24*(4), 310-320.

In: Thoracic Lymphadenopathy
Editor: Vikas Pathak

ISBN: 978-1-53616-700-9
© 2020 Nova Science Publishers, Inc.

Chapter 8

MISCELLANEOUS DISORDERS AFFECTING THORACIC LYMPH NODES

Samer Taj-Eldin, MD
WakeMed Health and Hospitals, Raleigh, North Carolina, US

INTRODUCTION

Lymphadenopathy is a common radiographic finding in many thoracic diseases and may be caused by a variety of infectious, inflammatory and neoplastic conditions [1]. This review aims to describe the patterns and management of three diseases in immunocompetent patients which can cause mediastinal and hilar lymphadenopathy.

CASTLEMAN'S DISEASE

Castleman's disease is an uncommon, mainly benign, lymphoproliferative disorder of unknown etiology. The overall prevalence of the disease is estimated to be less than 1/100,000. Castleman's disease may be localized or multifocal. The former, also known as unicentric Castleman's disease (UCD), presents with few or no symptoms, so its diagnosis is made typically through incidental radiological findings. This is generally a disease of younger adults, with median age at presentation of approximately 35 years. On chest radiographs, it may appear as an incidental, rounded, solitary mediastinal or hilar mass with a differential diagnosis that includes thymoma, lymphoma, neurogenic tumor and bronchial adenoma. On CT, it usually manifests as a homogenous, noninvasive, large solitary mass with soft-tissue attenuation, most commonly in the mediastinum or hila [1].

Life expectancy is usually not changed following the diagnosis of unicentric Castleman's disease. However, patients with UCD are at increased risk of developing paraneoplastic pemphigus and lymphomas, which can both be fatal. It is also associated with autoimmune diseases including autoimmune hemolytic anemia, immune thrombocytopenia, and acquired factor VIII deficiency. Complete surgical resection of the involved lymph node(s) is almost always curative and is considered the gold standard approach for the treatment of unicentric Castleman's disease. Recurrences of UCD have been rarely reported and are usually related to incomplete initial resection or missed lymph nodes at initial evaluation. Following excision, patients are followed annually with PET/CT and laboratory studies, which include CBC, LDH, chemistries with liver and renal function, and quantitative immunoglobulins. Annual imaging may be discontinued after five years if the patients remain disease free.

Multicentric Castleman's disease (MCD) presents with inflammatory symptoms including fever, night sweats, weight loss and anemia. Currently, it is most commonly diagnosed in individuals infected with HIV-1, although it certainly can develop in immunocompetent individuals. MCD manifests itself with generalized lymphadenopathy. In patients with multifocal disease, thoracic imaging may show bilateral hilar and mediastinal enlargement of lymph nodes (1-3cm in diameter), as well as diffuse reticulonodular pulmonary infiltrations. However, radiological findings are not sufficiently reliable to establish a diagnosis of Castleman's disease, which requires histological confirmation.

Miscellaneous Disorders Affecting Thoracic Lymph Nodes

Approximately half of patients with multifocal Castleman's disease are caused by HHV-8 (Human Herpes Virus) infection in human immunodeficiency virus (HIV)-positive or otherwise immunocompromised individuals. It is critical to distinguish patients with HHV-8-associated MCD from those with HHV-8-negative MCD at the time of diagnosis as their management differs. HHV-8 negative MCD can co-occur with POEMS, a paraneoplastic syndrome characterized by polyneuropathy, organomegaly, endocrinopathy, a monoclonal immunoglobulin spike, and skin changes such as hypertrichosis, acrocyanosis and plethora, hemangioma/ telangiectasia, thickening, or hyperpigmentation. Castleman disease is a major criterion in the diagnosis of POEMS syndrome.

When treating MCD without POEMS, the treatment typically incorporates the anti-IL-6 monoclonal antibody siltuximab for most patients. Additional agents are added for patients with MCD who develop life-threatening complications such as respiratory failure, renal failure, liver failure, and/or pancytopenia. This approach has resulted in two-year overall survival and relapse-free survival rates of 94 to 95 percent and 79 to 85 percent, respectively. Siltuximab is preferred based on its benefit in the only randomized trial and its approval in the United States and Europe for this purpose. If siltuximab is not available, tocilizumab, a monoclonal antibody targeted against the IL-6 receptor, can be used in its place.

When treating MCD with POEMS, the treatment depends on the number of bone lesions and whether clonal plasma cells are found on iliac crest biopsy. For patients with one to two isolated bone lesion(s) and without clonal plasma cells found on iliac crest biopsy, radiation to the affected site(s) is recommended. Patients are then followed annually with imaging (e.g., FDG PET/CT) and biomarkers. For patients with >2 bone lesions and/or with clonal plasma cells found on iliac crest biopsy, treatment approach depends on whether the patient is a candidate for an autologous hematopoietic cell transplantation (HCT). If the patient is an HCT candidate, then the suggested treatment is alkylator-based therapy; cyclophosphamide-based therapy; or two cycles of lenalidomide and dexamethasone, each followed by autologous HCT. If the patient is not an HCT candidate, the recommended treatment is either nine cycles of dexamethasone followed by 12 cycles of single agent lenalidomide or bortezomib/ cyclophosphamide/dexamethasone.

The natural history of HHV-8-negative/idiopathic MCD (iMCD) is variable. Several different patterns of disease progression have been described. An indolent form sometimes persists for months to a few years without worsening. An episodic relapsing form may be aggressive for a short period and then remit spontaneously or in response to treatment, only to recur at a later time. A rapidly progressive form that can lead to death within weeks. The prognosis of untreated MCD is poor. Few studies have investigated overall survival of MCD cases alone. Four large series reported overall survival for HIV-negative, likely-HHV-8-negative MCD cases. Five-year overall survival ranges from 55 to 77 percent.

LYMPHOMATOID GRANULOMATOSIS

Lymphomatoid Granulomatosis is a relatively rare pulmonary parenchymal disease characterized by angiocentric lymphoreticular proliferation and granulomatous disease [2]. It is thought to be an Epstein-Barr virus–associated systemic angiodestructive lymphoproliferative disease. It is characterized by prominent pulmonary involvement but can also involve multiple extrapulmonary sites. While the age range is from childhood to 80 years, most patients are 30 - 60 years old. Cough and pleuritic pain are the most common presenting symptoms. It can mimic Wegener Granulomatosis both clinically and radiographically.

The pathogenesis of lymphomatoid granulomatosis is unknown; however, recent studies have provided overwhelming evidence that lymphomatoid granulomatosis is a distinctive type of malignant B-cell lymphoma associated with immunosuppression. Scientific advances using flow cytometry and polymerase chain reaction (PCR) have allowed definitive cell phenotyping and assessment for T-cell receptor and immunoglobulin clonality, the hallmark of hematological malignancy. Surprisingly, these techniques have revealed that in most cases the large atypical cells represent malignant B cells and the T-cell component represents a prominent, polyclonal, reactive, T-cell infiltrate. It is best viewed as a T cell–rich, B-cell lymphoma.

Recent studies using a combination of PCR and in situ hybridization show that most lymphomatoid granulomatosis cases have malignant B cells containing Epstein-Barr virus (EBV) RNA. The biology of EBV infection involves binding to the complement receptor CD21 on B cells, resulting in the continuous growth or immortalization of infected B cells in vitro. In vivo, polyclonal, B-cell proliferation occurs, but it usually is controlled by immune regulation involving cytotoxic T cells. In immunodeficient states, the host's defenses may be unable to curb EBV-induced B-cell proliferation. In this regard, lymphomatoid granulomatosis shares characteristics with EBV-associated posttransplant lymphoma.

Establishing the diagnosis of lymphomatoid granulomatosis usually requires an open lung or video-assisted thoracoscopic biopsy. Transbronchial lung biopsy has not been studied rigorously. Because of the focal nature of lymphomatoid granulomatosis and the fact that it is not bronchocentric, a low diagnostic yield with bronchoscopic transbronchial biopsies is likely. In one study, the diagnosis was established with the aid of open lung biopsy in 70% of cases, bronchoscopic lung biopsy in 15% of cases, and extrapulmonary biopsy in 15% of cases [3]. In cases where bronchoscopic lung biopsy is nondiagnostic, a thoracoscopic lung biopsy may be necessary.

The therapeutic approach and optimal management have not been well defined. In several studies, therapy has ranged from observation to treatment with prednisone or chemotherapy. In the largest reported study of 152 patients, no significant difference in mortality or disease-free survival was found in treatment options, and the mortality rate exceeded 50%. New therapeutic approaches are necessary. In general, therapy for symptomatic or progressive disease involves prednisone with antineoplastic agents (e.g., Cyclophosphamide). Localized disease may respond to radiotherapy. In view of the association of lymphomatoid granulomatosis (LYG) with EBV and the similarity to posttransplant lymphoma, the use of antiviral drugs with minimal immunosuppressive therapy is advocated. Treatment options include ganciclovir, interferon alpha-2, or depending on histologic grade, combination chemotherapy [4].

In regards to prognosis, the median survival from diagnosis is 14 months. More than 60% of patients die within 5 years. The cause of death is usually extensive destruction of the pulmonary parenchyma, resulting in respiratory failure, sepsis, and, occasionally, massive hemoptysis. Poor prognostic indicators include an age younger than 30 years, neurological or hepatic involvement, leukopenia or pancytopenia.

ANGIOIMMUNOBLASTIC LYMPHADENOPATHY (AILD)

This disease is considered a systemic disorder resembling lymphoma characterized by fever, night sweats, weight loss, generalized lymphadenopathy, hepatosplenomegaly, maculopapular rash, polyclonal hypergammaglobulinemia, and Coombs-positive hemolytic anemia. This illness was initially considered to be a nonmalignant hyperimmune reaction to chronic antigenic stimulation; there is a proliferation of B-cells accompanied by profound deficiency of T cells. The disease follows a progressive but extremely variable course: some patients survive for a long period without chemotherapy; in other patients, overwhelming infections rapidly lead to death.

Recently it has been realized that essentially all cases of AILD have clonal rearrangements of T cell receptor genes and represent a frank T cell lymphoma rather than a benign entity with high risk for transformation to one. Moreover, genomic sequencing has revealed the presence of acquired "driver" mutations in genes previously linked to the pathogenesis of other hematologic cancers. For this reason, most medical specialists now use the term Angioimmunoblastic T-Cell Lymphoma (AILT) in describing this illness rather than AILD.

The most common chest radiographic finding is mediastinal lymphadenopathy. Alveolar shadows mimicking consolidation with or without pleural effusion may also be present. Pericardial involvement is also documented. The most common cause of death is opportunistic lung infections either due to pseudomonas, cytomegalovirus, Pneumocystis carinii or interstitial pneumonitis due to unknown etiology [5].

Morphologically, the involved lymph nodes demonstrate complete effacement of the normal architecture, prominent neovascularization and infiltration by immunoblasts and plasma cells. Other terms that have been used to describe this entity include diffuse plasmacytic sarcomatosis, immunoblastic lymphadenopathy, lymphogranulomatosis X, and immunologic aberrations in idiopathic reticulosis. Initially, AILD was thought to be a disease of B-cell origin that represented reactive immune response to unknown stimulus and high potential for malignant transformation. It is now evident that AILD in 80% of cases follows an aggressive course with short median survival, especially, if complete response with chemotherapy is not achieved. Despite the numerous reports on the role of Epstein-Barr virus in this disorder, it is unknown whether the presence of this virus is associated with the immune defect that accompanies AILD, or whether it is a pathogenetic factor. In contrast to non-Hodgkin's lymphomas, a stage is not usually assigned to the patient since the disease is systemic in nature, subsequently, parameters such as extent of disease and tumor bulk used to identify high-risk patients with non-Hodgkin's lymphomas, do not appear to correlate with disease activity or prognosis in AILD.

Treatment of AILD has been unsatisfactory, with approximately 25% of patients achieving complete and sustained remission when combined chemotherapy agents are used [6].

REFERENCES

[1] Nin, C. S. et al. *Respiratory Medicine*, 112 (2016): 10 – 17.
[2] Feigin, et al. *Am. J. Roentgenol.*, 129: 221 - 228; August 1977.
[3] Katzenstein, et al. Lymphomatoid granulomatosis: a clinicopathologic study of 152 cases. *Cancer*, 1979 Jan. 43(1):360 - 73.
[4] Rao et al. Lymphomatoid granulomatosis treated with rituximab and chemotherapy. *Clin. Adv. Hematol. Oncol.*, 2003 Nov. 1(11):658 - 60.

[5] Singh et al. Angioimmunoblastic Lymphadenopathy with Dysproteinemia: Thoracic Involvement; *Indian J. Chest Allied Sci.*, 2004; 46: 125 - 128.

[6] Sallah et al. Angioimmmunoblastic lymphadenopathy with dysproteinemia; emphasis on pathogenesis and treatment: *Acta Haemotology,* 1998: 99: 57 - 64.

In: Thoracic Lymphadenopathy
Editor: Vikas Pathak

ISBN: 978-1-53616-700-9
© 2020 Nova Science Publishers, Inc.

Chapter 9

ROLE OF EBUS/EUS IN THE DIAGNOSIS OF MEDIASTINAL AND HILAR LYMPHADENOPATHY

Raju Bishwakarma Century[1], MD
and Vikas Pathak[2], MD
[1]Winchester Medical Center, Winchester, Virginia, US
[2]Riverside Regional Medical Center, Newport News, Virginia, US

INTRODUCTION

Thoracic lymphadenopathy has broad differentials ranging from benign to malignant etiologies, making accurate diagnosis challenging. Although radiological evaluation with CT, MRI, or PET scan can aid in narrowing the differentials, their lack of specificity ultimately mandates tissue confirmation to establish a final diagnosis.

There are various options for tissue sampling such as mediastinoscopy, video-assisted thoracoscopic surgery (VATS) and minimally invasive approach such as transbronchial needle aspiration (TBNA), transthoracic needle aspiration (TTNA), endoscopic ultrasound guided fine needle aspiration (EUS- FNA) and endobronchial ultrasound guided transbronchial needle aspiration (EBUS -TBNA). In the current era, EBUS-TBNA has been widely used in the evaluation of mediastinal adenopathy, nodule or mass. Selection of each procedure depends on operators' skills, availability in practice, cost and patient preferences.

LYMPH NODE MAP

The most common lymph node mapping system currently used is the one developed by International Association for the Study of Lung Cancer (IASLC) in 2009 [1, 2, 3].

IASLC reconciled the old lymph node mapping system and proposed a new system with clear anatomic boundaries radiologically. IASLC system has created consistency in lung cancer staging and has improved communication among the providers taking care of patients with lung cancer. IASLC divides thoracic lymph nodes into seven zones and 14 stations [1, 3]. Station 1-9 are mediastinal lymph nodes and 10-14 are extra mediastinal lymph nodes. It is essential to understand anatomical boundaries of lymph node stations along with endoscopic landmarks for correctly identifying lymph nodes during EBUS or EUS [4-6]. EBUS can access lymph nodes stations 2, 4, 7, 10 and 11 and EUS can access lymph node stations 4L, 7, 8 9 and liver and adrenal metastasis [6].

Supraclavicular Zone

Station 1

Supraclavicular lymph nodes are station 1 lymph nodes. The upper border is the lower margin of cricoid cartilage. The lower border is the upper border of manubrium. The midline of the trachea divides the 1R lymph node from the 1L lymph node. Station 1 lymph nodes are not easily located with EBUS due to their superior location [3].

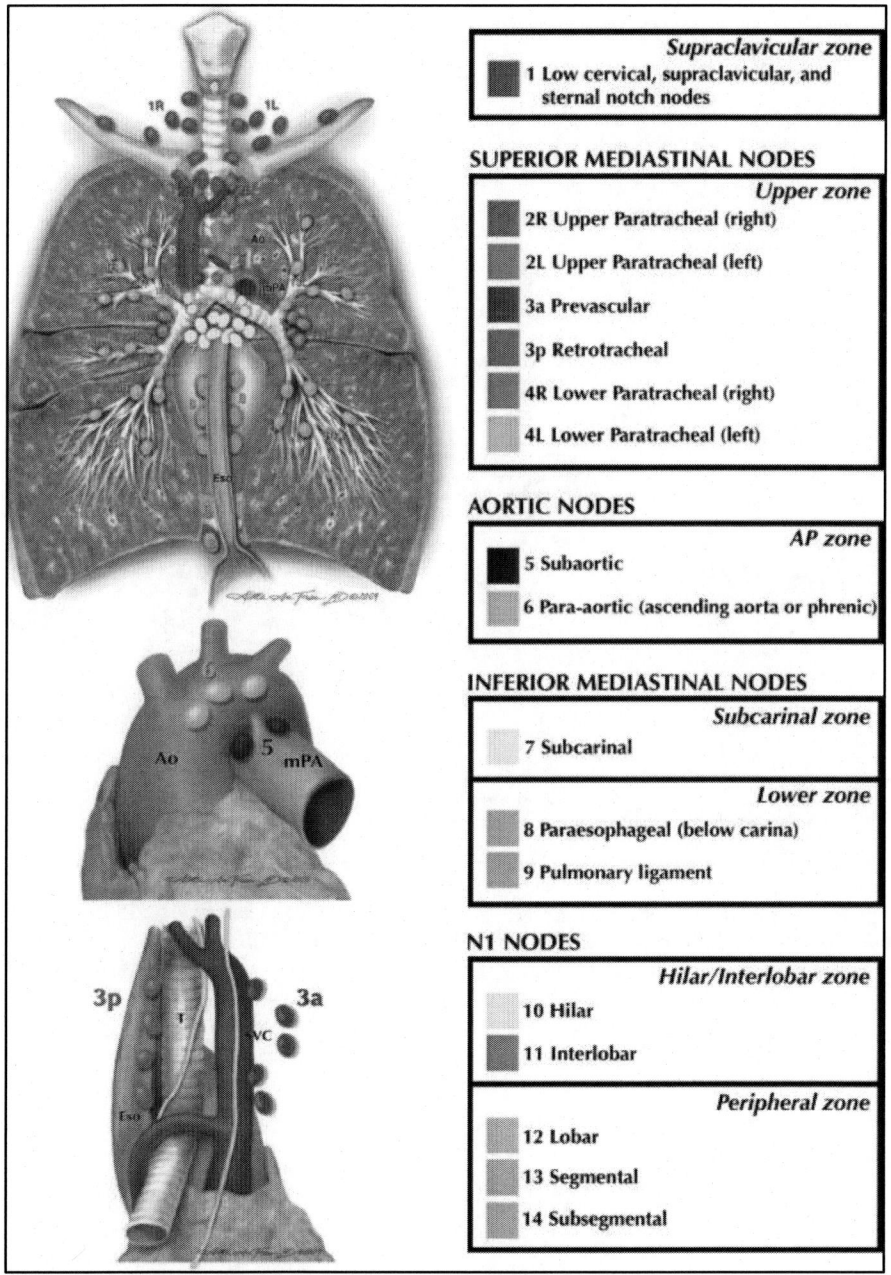

Figure 1. The International Association for the Study of Lung Cancer (IASLC) lymph node map, including the proposed grouping of lymph node stations into "zones" for the purposes of prognostic analyses (Image reproduced with permission from IASLC).

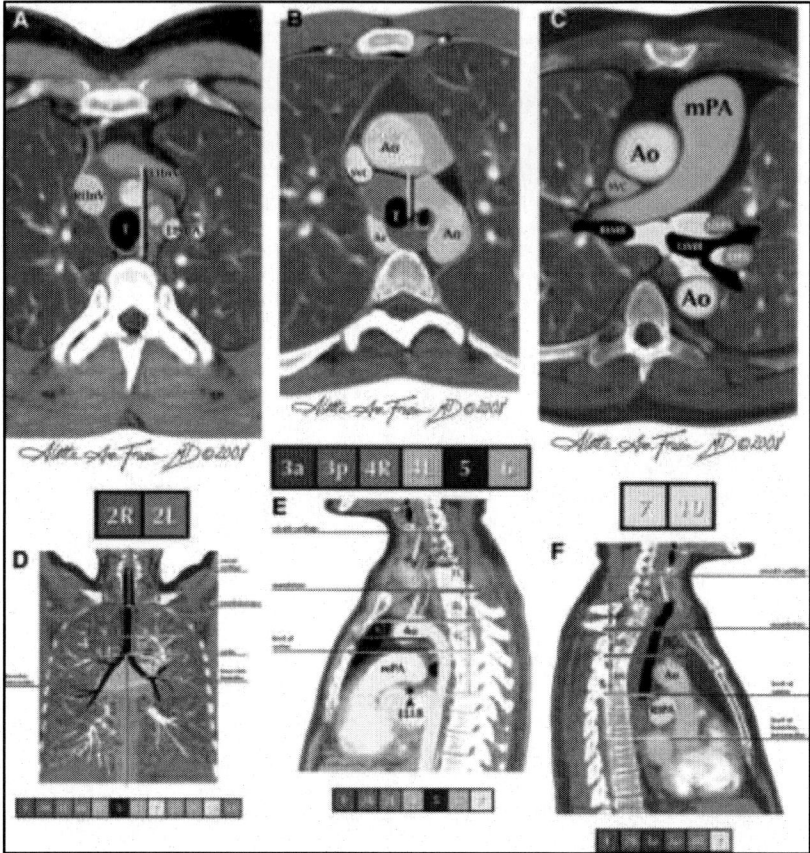

Figure 2. The International Association for the Study of Lung Cancer (IASLC) lymph node map, including the proposed grouping of lymph node stations into "zones" for the purposes of prognostic analyses (Image reproduced with permission from IASLC).

Upper Zone

Station 2

Station 2 consists of the upper paratracheal lymphnodes. The right upper border (2R) landmarks are the apex of right lung and pleural space. The upper border in the midline is the upper border of manubrium. The right lower border is the intersection of innominate vein with trachea. The upper border landmarks for the left (2L) correspond to 2R with apex of lung and the upper border of manubrium. The lower border consists of the superior border of the aortic arch [1, 3]. The innominate vein on the right and the aortic arch on left separate 2R from 4R, and 2L from 4L, respectively [7, 8]. Unlike 1R and 1L, 2R and 2L are separated by the left lateral border of the trachea (not the midline of the trachea) [1, 3].

Station 3

Station 3 lymph nodes are perivascular lymph nodes, which are further divided into anterior (3A) and posterior (3P). The upper border is marked by the thoracic inlet and the lower margin by the carina. The anterior border of 3A is the sternum, while the posterior border is superior vena cava (SVC) [1]. Posterior 3P is located between the trachea anteriorly and vertebrae posteriorly [1]. EBUS can visualize 3A and 3P lymph nodes well, but it is technically difficult to obtain aspiration through EBUS –TBNA [8] due to its location.

Station 4

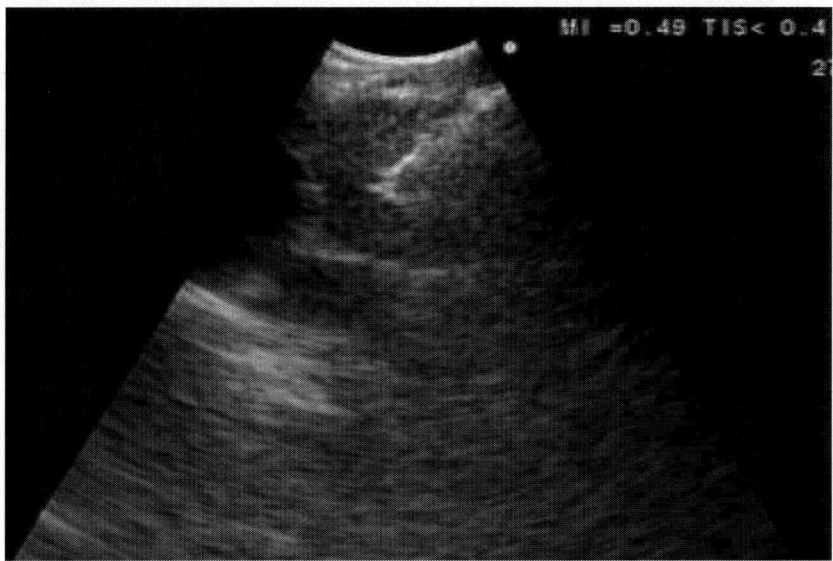

Figure 3. Station 4 R lymph node with needle into the lymph node.

Lower paratracheal lymph nodes are station 4R and 4L. The upper border of 4R is the intersection of the caudal margin of innominate vein with trachea, and lower border is the lower border of azygos vein [1]. EBUS can localize both the brachiocephalic and azygos vein [7, 8]. Posterior landmarks of 4R are the SVC and aorta. The left border of trachea separates between 4R and 4L. The 4L located in aortopulmonary window between two large vascular structure aorta and left pulmonary artery. The upper border is the lower margin of aortic arch and lower border is the upper rim of left pulmonary artery [1]. Both EBUS and EUS can access the 4L lymph node [8].

Aortopulmonary Zone

Station 5

Aortopulmonary or subaortic lymph nodes are station 5. The upper border is the lower border of aortic arch and the lower border is the upper border of left pulmonary artery but lateral to ligamentum arteriosum. Station 4 and 5 are separated by ligamentum arteriosum [1]. Transvascular approach has been attempted to access station 5 by puncturing pulmonary artery [9].

Station 6

Paraaortic lymph nodes are station 6, located anterolateral to the aortic arch and ascending aorta. The upper border is a tangential line to the upper border of aortic arch and lower border is by the lower border of aortic arch [1]. EBUS and EUS can occasionally visualize station 6 lymph nodes but aspiration is not possible. However, sampling station 6 LN has been attempted by vascular puncture via transaortic approach [9, 10].

Subcarinal Zone

Station 7

Subcarinal lymph nodes are station 7. The upper border is the carina. The right lower border is the lower border of bronchus intermedius and left lower border is determined by the upper border of left lower bronchus [1, 3]. EBUS can approach station 7 from either right or left mainstem bronchi. EUS can visualize station 7 between the left atrium and right pulmonary artery for EUS-FNA. [5, 7, 8].

Lower Zone

Station 8

Station 8 are the paraoesophageal lymph nodes, which cannot c be visualized by EBUS. The upper border on right side is marked by the lower border of bronchus intermedius and left upper border is upper border of the left lower bronchus. The midline separates 8L from 8R [1, 3]. Lower border on both sides is marked by the diaphragm [7]. EUS can visualize and sample station 8 via EUS –FNA [8, 5].

Station 9

Pulmonary ligament lymph nodes constitute station 9, which is located between the inferior pulmonary vein and the diaphragm within in pulmonary ligament [1]. Station 9 cannot be visualized or accessed by EBUS, but can be by EUS for EUS-FNA [8].

EXTRA-MEDIASTINAL NODES

Hilar Zone

Station 10

Station 10 are comprised of hilar lymph nodes. The upper border of 10R is the lower border of azygos vein and the upper border of 10 L is upper border of the left pulmonary artery. The lower border bilaterally is the interlobar region [1]. EBUS can easily localize the vascular landmark and bronchoscopically it is immediately adjacent to main stem bronchus [7, 8]. Station 10 is inaccessible by EUS [8].

Station 11

Interlobar lymph nodes are station 11R and 11L. Station 11R is further divided into 11Rs, which is between the upper lobe to the bronchus intermedius, and 11Ri, which is between the middle lobe and lower lobe [1, 3]. These lymph nodes are also only accessible by EBUS but not EUS [8].

Peripheral Zones

Station 12 lymph nodes are adjacent to the lobar bronchi
Station 13 lymph nodes are adjacent to the segmental bronchi
Station 14 lymph nodes are adjacent to the subsegmental bronchi.

Lymph nodes are further classified into N1, N2 and N3 regional groups as per the TNM system in reference to tumor location. N1 refers to lymph node metastasis to an ipsilateral hilar or peripheral zone lymph node. N2 refers to lymph node metastasis to an ipsilateral mediastinal lymph node and/or metastasis to a subcarinal lymph node. N3 refers to lymph node metastasis to a contralateral mediastinal, hilar or peripheral zone, or to an ipsilateral or contralateral low cervical or supraclavicular lymph node [3].

ENDOBRONCHIAL ULTRASOUND GUIDED TRANSBRONCHIAL NEEDLE ASPIRATION (EBUS-TBNA)

There are two kinds of EBUS. Radial EBUS and linear probe or convex probe EBUS. Radial EBUS is primarily used in the evaluation of peripheral lesion. It has been used for real-time localization of mediastinal lymph nodes during conventional transbronchial needle biopsy. Convex probe or linear EBUS has replaced radial EBUS in the evaluation of mediastinal and hilar adenopathy. In the recent era, EBUS-TBNA is preferred over other methods in the invasive mediastinal staging of lung cancer [11].

Convex probe EBUS has an ultrasound probe attached at the end of flexible bronchoscope. EBUS made it possible to visualize the bronchoscopic view of airway and the sonographic view of a lymph node simultaneously. It is equipped with capabilities to measure the size, study the shape and, characterize the echotexture. Doppler capability made it possible to study the vascularity and vascular structure around the lymph node.

Techniques

EBUS can be performed in different settings and locations depending on the operators' comfort, skills and availability of resources. It can be performed in bronchoscopy suite or operating room, under either conscious moderate sedation or deep sedation [12]. Studies have shown that there is no significant difference in safety or sample yield between types of anesthesia [13, 14]. However, a few studies showed deep sedation is associated with shorter procedure times, increased numbers of lymph nodes, and access to smaller lymph nodes [15, 16]. The bronchoscopist must consider skill sets, local resources and patient factors such as pulmonary reserve and comorbidities to choose the optimal modality of anesthesia and location [12, 13].

Deep sedation, or general anesthesia, requires airway and ventilatory support either via laryngeal mask airway (LMA) or endotracheal tube (ETT). Usually LMA size 4 and 5 or ET tube size 8 is necessary to accomadate the EBUS scope [12, 17]. ET tube approximation to the tracheal wall can make accessing the paratracheal lymph nodes challenging. It may be necessary to withdraw the ET tube slightly in order to expose the upper paratracheal lymph nodes [12, 17].

During the mediastinum survey, lymph node morphology can be studied before a needle biopsy. EBUS is equipped to study size, shape, sonographic echogenicity, vascularity, and adjacent vascular structure. Sonographic characteristics are useful to differentiate between benign vs malignant nature of a lymph node. Round shape, central necrosis, size >1 cm and increased vascularity are more likely to be malignant. If the lymph node is round, has a distinct margin, is heterogeneous and has central necrosis, it has apositive predictive value of being malignant of approximately 60% [17, 18].

However, lymph node characteristics are not reliable in differentiating malignant vs. benign disease and therefore, irrespective of feature, all lymph nodes should be sampled. In case of negative biopsy, malignant appearing lymph node should be considered to biopsy by alternative methods. Newer sonographic feature such as elastography properties is being studied to differentiate benign vs. malignant disease depending on color characteristics [18].

After localization of a lymph node, sampling is done by transbronchial needle aspiration. The lymph node is aspirated in real time under direct visualization by transbronchial needle. The transbronchial needle has different parts, such as the handle, needle stopper, and sheath adjuster. Needle has sheath outside and stylet inside. Once the targeted lymph node is identified, TBNA needle is introduced via the working channel and locked in place. The needle sheath should be adjusted just enough to see at the tip of the bronchoscope. After finding the target, advance the needle to puncture the target under the direct visualization. After puncturing, the stylet is removed, and needle aspiration performed to obtain lymphoid tissues. Aspiration is obtained by agitation of needle ranging from 5-15times. Usually 3-5 passes are necessary from each lymph node in order to obtain an adequate sample [17].

There are various methods of obtaining needle aspiration such as using negative pressure suction, capillary suction without needle or aspiration by partial retraction of the stylet. None of the methods are found to be superior to each other or to improve diagnostic yield [17]. EBUS-TBNA using either capillary sampling or complete stylet removal are effective and has a high proportion of satisfactory results for ancillary testing [19]. Commonly used TBNA needle are 21 gauge and 22 gauge and others are 19-gauge flex needle or smaller 25-gauge needle. Multiple studies showed that diagnostic yield is similar between different needle sizes [17, 20]. Few studies suggested that flexible 19-gauge nitinol needle has some improvement in diagnostic yield. Flexible nature of this needle could facilitate better access to lymph node station 4L and 10 L lymph nodes [21]. Besides the techniques and tools, other factors for lower diagnostic yield are lymph nodes less than 5mm, distorted airway, paratracheal location, and calcified lymph nodes [22].

After tissues are obtained from needle aspiration, a cytotechnologist or a cytopathologist evaluate the air fixed cell with "diff quick" stain immediately in the procedure room for Rapid On-Site Evaluation (ROSE). ROSE provides information to bronchoscopist about adequacy of sampling, triaging specimen for ancillary test and provide preliminary diagnosis. Studies found no difference in diagnostic yield or procedure time. However, ROSE was associated with fewer needle passes, lower complication rates and lower additional bronchoscopic procedures. [17, 23]. EBUS-TBNA specimens are adequate for molecular analysis [17, 24]. In a seven-year-audit, Stevenson found EBUS with ROSE increases yield for molecular testing [24, 25]. EBUS-TBNA with ROSE is also associated with ensuring a qualified specimen, thereby improving diagnostic rate and reducing complications [26]. EBUS-ROSE allows immediate processing and interpretation which eventually translates into lower costs compared to conventional EBUS without ROSE [27]. As the importance of ROSE is becoming increasingly evident, telecytology for ROSE could be a pivotal tool in a resource-limited health center [24].

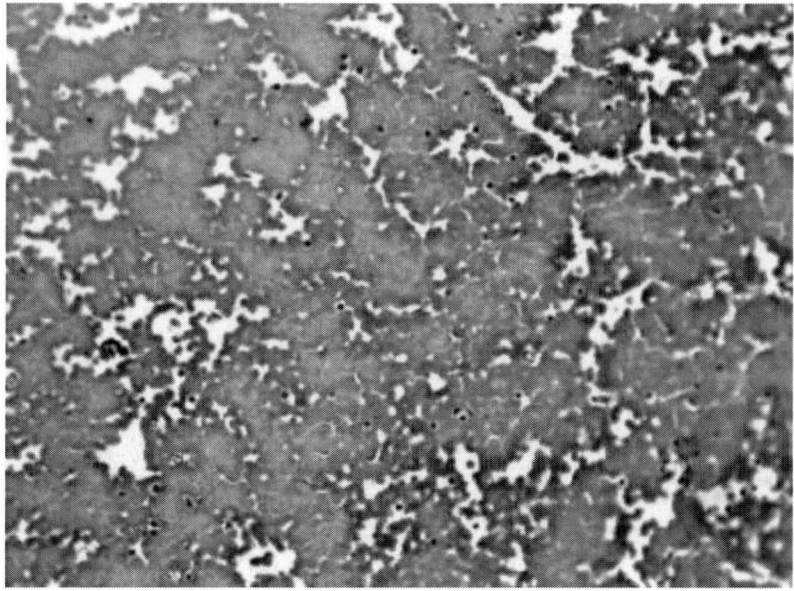

Figure 4. Diff quick stain from EBUS-TBNA showing lymphocytes and blood.

EUS-FNA is performed with similar set up and techniques. EUS has linear ultrasound at the tip of the endoscope and can evaluate the mediastinum through the esophagus. Since the airway does not need to be involved, EUS can be better tolerated than EBUS. Similar to EBUS, EUS-FNA utilizes similar needles (21-22 gauge), aspiration techniques, and processing with ROSE [28].

ROLE OF EBUS IN DIAGNOSIS AND STAGING OF LUNG CANCER

Lung cancer was the leading cause of cancer death in the world in 2018. Lung cancer is not the most common in woman, however, it is rising. In 28 countries, lung cancer is the leading cause of death in both genders [29]. Overall, prognosis of lung cancer has been poor. Early detection of lung cancer and precision medicine with targeted therapy has improved overall prognosis and survival [30]. Correct staging of lung cancer is the cornerstone for accurate communication among physicians, formulation of a treatment plan, and prognostication of survival [11]. The nodal station is essential in TNM staging of lung cancer. Nodal staging is recommended in non-small cell lung cancer and limited stage small cell cancer. Radiological staging is done by CT or PET scan, but invasive staging is essential to confirm lymph node metastasis.

CT scan is the initial investigation of choice, providing location of suspicious lesion(s) and identifying mediastinal involvement. In general, lymph node size >1cm is considered lymphadenopathy. CT characteristics of lymph nodes cannot be reliable in clinical staging. The sensitivity and specificity on detecting lymph node metastases by CT are 55% and 81% respectively [11]. PET scan is more accurate than CT scan on detecting lymph node metastases. PET scan utilizes the metabolic activity but its sensitivity decreases with size <7-10 mm [11]. PET scan can be falsely positive due to infection and inflammation. Hence, PET positive lymph node needs further tissue confirmation. PET scan median sensitivity and specificity on detecting lymph node metastasis is 80% and 88%, respectively [11].

Centrally located tumor, size more than 3 cm, and involvement of N1 lymph nodes are high risk for mediastinal disease, and should go for invasive staging irrespective of lymph node size or PET positivity. Even in the absence of radiographically abnormal mediastinal lymph nodes, the prevalence of mediastinal (N2/N3) involvement consistently exceeds 10% in tumors with high-risk features for mediastinal disease [11, 31]. Despite its importance, invasive staging is still underutilized. Osarogiagbon study showed that 63% of patients with high risk for nodal metastasis did not undergo invasive staging [32, 33,34].

Invasive mediastinal staging can be surgical or minimally invasive via needle aspiration. Surgical techniques are cervical mediastinoscopy, anterior mediastinotomy, and video assisted thoracoscopic surgery (VATS). Minimally invasive procedure options are transbronchial needle aspiration (TBNA), transthoracic needle aspiration (TTNA) and EBUS-TBNA or EUS-TBNA. In the current era, EBUS is the most preferable method for invasive staging [11, 17]. EBUS can sample lymph node stations 2, 4, 7, 10 and 11, but cannot sample 5,6,8 and 9. Cervical mediastinoscopy is preferred invasive alternative methods for negative EBUS-TBNA. The median sensitivity for EBUS-TBNA is 89%, with values ranging from 46% to 97% and the median negative predicted value is 91% [11].

There is significant heterogenicity in practice of EBUS in lung cancer staging. EBUS-TBNA can be performed to sample radiologically abnormal lymph node or systematically stage by starting from highest N3 nodes. Miller et al. found that 74% of bronchoscopist start staging from N3 hilar nodes [31]. Lymph node sampling should be systematic, starting from highest N3, followed by N2 and N1. Lymph nodes more than 5 mm and at least three N2/N3 nodes should be sampled to increase the sensitivity and negative predictive value [35].

ROLE OF EUS-FNA IN LUNG CANCER

EBUS-TBNA can access mediastinal and hilar lymph nodes except stations 5,6,8 and 9. EUS- FNA can sample station 4L, 7, 8 and 9 lymph nodes [28]. The median sensitivity and specificity is 89% and 100%, respectively [11, 28]. EUS also visualized left adrenal and left lobe of liver and therefore can assist to stage distant metastasis to liver and adrenal glands [28]. EUS-FNA is complimentary to EBUS-TBNA to access inaccessible areas by EBUS. Combining EUS and EBUS increases specificity, negative and positive predictive value. EUS can be considered when EBUS-TBNA is negative, before going for an invasive staging procedure. Negative predictive value of combined EUS/EBUS is 100% when a mediastinal lymph node is more than1 cm on PET/CT and 94% when a mediastinal lymph node is less than 1 cm [28].

EUS performed by gastroenterologist and EBUS-TBNA by pulmonologist. Some of the interventional pulmonologists are trained for both and can do both procedures at the same time. Team approach with gastroenterologist and pulmonologist can perform EUS and EBUS in same set up for complete mediastinum staging.

ROLE OF EBUS IN MEDIASTINAL TUMOR AND EXTRA THORACIC MALIGNANCY

Besides the primary lung cancer, mediastinal and hilar adenopathy can be seen in lymphoma and metastasis from extra thoracic malignancies. Both non-Hodgkin lymphoma (NHL) and Hodgkin disease (HD) lymphoma can involve the thorax. Non-Hodgkin lymphoma usually involve 40-50% and HD about 85% [36]. Hodgkin disease usually involves pre-vascular and paratracheal lymph nodes and NHL involve subcarinal, paraoesophageal and internal mammary lymph nodes. Tissues confirmation is important to differentiate between specific types of lymphoma [37, 38]. Diagnostic accuracies of EBUS-TBNA is variable and pooled diagnostic accuracy is

68%. Samples in recurrent lymphoma has a higher yield than de novo lymphoma [17]. Dhooria et al. found sensitivity of EBUS-TBNA in new onset and recurrent lymphomas 72.7% and 73.3%, respectively, and 24% were adequately subtyped [39]. Sensitivity, specificity and negative predictive value were 100%, 100% and 96% respectively, by combining ROSE and flow cytometry [40]. Despite variable accuracies and conflicting evidence, EBUS is minimally invasive and has a good safety profile. EBUS-TBNA should be considered first to evaluate in suspected lymphoma [17].

Extra-thoracic malignancy such as breast, head and neck, gastrointestinal, and genitourinary can metastasize to mediastinal lymph nodes. Other benign and malignant tumors can present as mediastinal masses such as thymoma, lipoma, neurogenic tumors, thymic carcinoma and benign cysts [41]. There is discordance between PET positivity and lymph node metastases in extra thoracic malignancy. Mehta, etal showed that about 70% of PET-positive lymph nodes were benign [42]. EBUS has high diagnostic accuracy in diagnosis of intrathoracic lymph node metastasis from extra-thoracic malignancies [42-44]. The overall pooled sensitivity and specificity ranges from 85 - 86% and 98-100%, respectively [43].

ROLE OF EBUS IN GRANULOMATOUS LYMPHADENITIS

Granulomatous inflammation of mediastinal lymph node is associated with malignancies, inflammatory conditions such sarcoidosis, silicosis, berylliosis, drug induced, hypersensitivity pneumonitis, Crohn's disease and various infections like tuberculosis, histoplasmosis, and coccidiomycosis [45, 46]. Clinical, histological, endemic geographical location, other concomitant diseases, and other supportive laboratory data should be considered to make a diagnosis of a granulomatous condition.

Sarcoidosis

Sarcoidosis is a systemic granulomatous inflammatory condition primarily affecting the lung. Pulmonary sarcoidosis classified in 5 stages by radiological features. Stage 0: No sign of granulomas in the lungs or lymph nodes; Stage 1: Bilateral hilar lymphadenopathy; Stage 2: Bilateral hilar adenopathy with pulmonary infiltrates; Stage 3: Pulmonary infiltrates only without adenopathy; Stage 4: Pulmonary fibrosis [47]. Right Paratracheal and bilateral hilar lymphadenopathy is commonest presentation. Unilateral hilar adenopathy is uncommon in 3-5% of sarcoidosis [48]. Mediastinal adenopathy without hilar adenopathy and anterior or posterior mediastinal adenopathy are unusual presentation and should raise caution on diagnosis [45]. Sarcoidosis in endemic area for tuberculosis, coccidioidomycosis and histoplasmosis can be challenging [45]. The diagnostic yield of EBUS-TBNA ranged from 54% to 93%, with the pooled diagnostic accuracy of 79% [17]. Diagnostic yield could vary with stages. Sun et al. showed that 98% yield with stage 1 as compared to 87% in stage II sarcoidosis [49]. However, Goyal et al. showed no correlation of clinical findings or radiological stages on diagnostic yield [48].

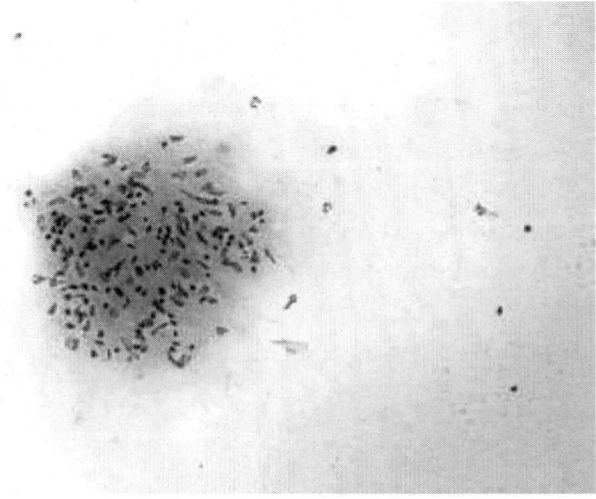

Image 5. Diff quick stain from sample obtained from EBUS-TBNA showing granuloma.

Tuberculosis

Tuberculosis is also known as "great mimicker" and can affect every organ system. Active tuberculosis could be primary or post primary tuberculosis. Mediastinal and hilar adenopathy is most frequent radiological presentation in primary tuberculosis [45, 50]. There is overlap between sarcoidosis and tuberculous lymph node cytology and morphology but extensive necrotizing granuloma is more common in tuberculosis [51]. Other supportive clinical and laboratory data should be considered such as endemic area, staining, PPD or Gold QuantiFERON tests along with molecular diagnostic test. Diagnosis is supported by clinical context, AFB staining and detection of genetic material in tissue [17, 45]. Overall diagnostic yield of EBUS-TBNA ranges from 80-84% [17, 52]. Eometal. showed overall increase in diagnostic accuracy of EBUS-TBNA to 94% when TB-PCR is combined with the histological and microbiological data [53].

FUNGAL INFECTION

Mediastinal adenopathy could be the initial presentation of fungal infections such as histoplasmosis and coccidioidomycosis. Mediastinal and hilar adenopathy is a common presentation in the acute form of the disease [45]. Granuloma can be necrotizing or non-necrotizing in fungal infection [54]. Fungal tissues culture, staining for fungal elements in tissues and serologies should be considered to improve diagnostic accuracy [54, 55]. Combined EBUS-TBNA and EUS-FNA are associated with early and accurate diagnosis of pulmonary coccidomycosis [56].

ROLE OF EBUS IN BENIGN LESION

Many other non-neoplastic, noninfectious conditions can cause enlargement of mediastinal lymph nodes such silicosis, drug reactions, amyloidosis, heart failure, Castleman's disease and chronic obstructive pulmonary disease (COPD) [45]. Evaluation of mediastinal adenopathy in the presence of multiple comorbidities could be challenging and warrants tissues confirmation. EBUS-TBNA and EUS-FNA are safe and minimally invasive approach for tissue confirmation of benign etiology.

REFERENCES

[1] Rusch, V. W., Asamura, H., Watanabe, H., Giroux, D. J., Rami-Porta, R., Goldstraw, P. The IASLC lung cancer staging project: a proposal for a new international lymph node map in the forthcoming seventh edition of the TNM classification for lung cancer. *J Thorac Oncol.* 2009;4(5):568-577.

[2] Kim, J. H., van Beek E, Jr., Murchison, J. T., Marin, A., Mirsadraee, S. The International Association for the Study of Lung Cancer Lymph Node Map: A Radiologic Atlas and Review. *Tuberculosis and respiratory diseases.* 2015;78(3):180-189.

[3] El-Sherief, A. H., Lau, C. T., Wu, C. C., Drake, R. L., Abbott, G. F., Rice, T. W. International association for the study of lung cancer (IASLC) lymph node map: radiologic review with CT illustration. *Radiographics.* 2014;34(6):1680-1691.

[4] Konge, L., Colella, S., Vilmann, P., Clementsen, P. F. How to learn and to perform endoscopic ultrasound and endobronchial ultrasound for lung cancer staging: A structured guide and review. *Endoscopic ultrasound.* 2015;4(1):4-9.

[5] Sharma, M., Pathak, A., Shoukat, A., Somani, P. Imaging of spaces of neck and mediastinum by endoscopic ultrasound. *Lung India : official organ of Indian Chest Society.* 2016;33(3):292-305.

[6] Jenssen, C., Annema, J. T., Clementsen, P., Cui, X-W., Borst, M. M., Dietrich, C. F. Ultrasound techniques in the evaluation of the mediastinum, part 2: mediastinal lymph node anatomy and diagnostic reach of ultrasound techniques, clinical work up of neoplastic and inflammatory mediastinal lymphadenopathy using ultrasound

techniques and how to learn mediastinal endosonography. *Journal of thoracic disease.* 2015;7(10):E439-E458.
[7] Yasufuku, K. EBUS-TBNA bronchoscopy. In: A. Ernst FH, ed. *Endobronchial ultrasound: An atlas and practical guide.* 2009:119-144.
[8] Tournoy, K. G., Annema, J. T., Krasnik, M., Herth, F. J., van Meerbeeck, J. P. Endoscopic and endobronchial ultrasonography according to the proposed lymph node map definition in the seventh edition of the tumor, node, metastasis classification for lung cancer. *J Thorac Oncol.* 2009;4(12):1576-1584.
[9] Kazakov, J., Hegde, P., Tahiri, M., Thiffault, V., Ferraro, P., Liberman, M. Endobronchial and Endoscopic Ultrasound-Guided Transvascular Biopsy of Mediastinal, Hilar, and Lung Lesions. *Ann Thorac Surg.* 2017;103(3):951-955.
[10] Bendzsak, A., Oliveira, R., Goudie, E., et al. Evaluation of the Mediastinum: Differentiating Between Stations 4L, 5, and 6 Using EBUS and EUS. *Ann Thorac Surg.* 2017;103(2):e219-e221.
[11] Silvestri, G. A., Gonzalez, A. V., Jantz, M. A., et al. Methods for staging non-small cell lung cancer: Diagnosis and management of lung cancer, 3rd ed: American College of Chest Physicians evidence-based clinical practice guidelines. *Chest.* 2013;143(5 Suppl):e211S-e250S.
[12] Canneto, B., Ferraroli, G., Falezza, G., Infante, M. V. Ideal conditions to perform EBUS-TBNA. *J Thorac Dis.* 2017;9(Suppl 5):S414-s417.
[13] Aswanetmanee, P., Limsuwat, C., Kabach, M., Alraiyes, A. H., Kheir, F. The role of sedation in endobronchial ultrasound-guided transbronchial needle aspiration: Systematic review. *Endosc Ultrasound.* 2016;5(5):300-306.
[14] Casal, R. F., Lazarus, D. R., Kuhl, K., et al. Randomized trial of endobronchial ultrasound-guided transbronchial needle aspiration under general anesthesia versus moderate sedation. *American journal of respiratory and critical care medicine.* 2015;191(7):796-803.
[15] Yarmus, L. B., Akulian, J. A., Gilbert, C., et al. Comparison of moderate versus deep sedation for endobronchial ultrasound

transbronchial needle aspiration. *Ann Am Thorac Soc.* 2013;10(2):121-126.

[16] Ost, D. E., Ernst, A., Lei, X., et al. Diagnostic yield of endobronchial ultrasound-guided transbronchial needle aspiration: results of the AQuIRE Bronchoscopy Registry. *Chest.* 2011;140(6):1557-1566.

[17] Wahidi, M. M., Herth, F., Yasufuku, K., et al. Technical Aspects of Endobronchial Ultrasound-Guided Transbronchial Needle Aspiration: CHEST Guideline and Expert Panel Report. *CHEST.* 2016;149(3):816-835.

[18] Dietrich, C. F., Jenssen, C., Herth FJF. Endobronchial ultrasound elastography. *Endoscopic ultrasound.* 2016;5(4):233-238.

[19] Fernandez-Bussy, S., Biswas, A., Labarca, G., Jantz, M. A., Mehta, H. J. Comparison of Endobronchial Ultrasound-guided Transbronchial Needle Aspiration With Stylet Retracted Partially Versus Completely for Molecular Testing. *J Bronchology Interv Pulmonol.* 2019;26(3):222-224.

[20] Chaddha, U., Ronaghi, R., Elatre, W., Chang, C. F., Mahdavi, R. Comparison of Sample Adequacy and Diagnostic Yield of 19- and 22-G EBUS-TBNA Needles. *J Bronchology Interv Pulmonol.* 2018;25(4):264-268.

[21] Tremblay, A., Hergott, C. A. 19-G EBUS: Why, When, and How? In: *J Bronchology Interv Pulmonol.* Vol 25. United States2018:257-259.

[22] Kennedy, M. P., Jimenez, C. A., Morice, R. C., et al. Factors Influencing the Diagnostic Yield of Endobronchial Ultrasound-guided Transbronchial Needle Aspiration. *J Bronchology Interv Pulmonol.* 2010;17(3):202-208.

[23] Sehgal, I. S., Dhooria, S., Aggarwal, A. N., Agarwal, R. Impact of Rapid On-Site Cytological Evaluation (ROSE) on the Diagnostic Yield of Transbronchial Needle Aspiration During Mediastinal Lymph Node Sampling: Systematic Review and Meta-Analysis. *Chest.* 2018;153(4):929-938.

[24] Jain, D., Allen, T. C., Aisner, D. L., et al. Rapid On-Site Evaluation of Endobronchial Ultrasound-Guided Transbronchial Needle Aspirations for the Diagnosis of Lung Cancer: A Perspective From Members of

the Pulmonary Pathology Society. *Arch Pathol Lab Med.* 2018;142(2):253-262.

[25] Stevenson, T., Powari, M., Bowles, C. Evolution of a rapid onsite evaluation (ROSE) service for endobronchial ultrasound guided (EBUS) fine needle aspiration (FNA) cytology in a UK Hospital: A 7 year audit. *Diagn Cytopathol.* 2018;46(8):656-662.

[26] Xiang, Q., Wan, T., Hu, Q., Chen, H., Li, D. [Value of C-ROSE During EBUS-TBNA to Obtain the Tissue Sample in the Diagnosis of Lung Cancer]. *Zhongguo Fei Ai Za Zhi.* 2018;21(11):833-840.

[27] Kalluri, M., Puttagunta, L., Ohinmaa, A., Thanh, N. X., Wong, E. Cost Analysis of Intra Procedural Rapid on Site Evaluation of Cytopathology With Endobronchial Ultrasound. *Int J Technol Assess Health Care.* 2015;31(5):273-280.

[28] Jue, T. L., Sharaf, R. N., Appalaneni, V., et al. Role of EUS for the evaluation of mediastinal adenopathy. *Gastrointest Endosc.* 2011;74(2):239-245.

[29] Latest global cancer data: Cancer burden rises to 18.1 million new cases and 9.6 million cancer deaths in 2018 [press release]. International Agency for Research On Cancer, WHO2018.

[30] Lou, Y., Dholaria, B., Soyano, A., et al. Survival trends among non-small-cell lung cancer patients over a decade: impact of initial therapy at academic centers. *Cancer Med.* 2018;7(10):4932-4942.

[31] Miller, R. J., Mudambi, L., Vial, M. R., Hernandez, M., Eapen, G. A. Evaluation of Appropriate Mediastinal Staging among Endobronchial Ultrasound Bronchoscopists. *Ann Am Thorac Soc.* 2017;14(7):1162-1168.

[32] Liam, C. K., Andarini, S., Lee, P., Ho, J. C., Chau, N. Q., Tscheikuna, J. Lung cancer staging now and in the future. *Respirology.* 2015;20(4):526-534.

[33] Osarogiagbon, R. U., Lee, Y. S., Faris, N. R., Ray, M. A., Ojeabulu, P. O., Smeltzer, M. P. Invasive mediastinal staging for resected non-small cell lung cancer in a population-based cohort. *J Thorac Cardiovasc Surg.* 2019.

[34] Czarnecka-Kujawa, K., Yasufuku, K. The role of endobronchial ultrasound versus mediastinoscopy for non-small cell lung cancer. *Journal of thoracic disease.* 2017;9(Suppl 2):S83-S97.

[35] Evison, M., Crosbie, P., Navani, N., et al. How should performance in EBUS mediastinal staging in lung cancer be measured? In: *Br J Cancer.* Vol 115. England2016:e9.

[36] Bligh, M. P., Borgaonkar, J. N., Burrell, S. C., MacDonald, D. A., Manos, D. Spectrum of CT Findings in Thoracic Extranodal Non-Hodgkin Lymphoma. *Radiographics.* 2017;37(2):439-461.

[37] Bae, Y. A., Lee, K. S. Cross-sectional evaluation of thoracic lymphoma. *Thorac Surg Clin.* 2010;20(1):175-186.

[38] Thomas, A. G., Vaidhyanath, R., Kirke, R., Rajesh, A. Extranodal lymphoma from head to toe: part 2, the trunk and extremities. *AJR Am J Roentgenol.* 2011;197(2):357-364.

[39] Dhooria, S., Mehta, R. M., Madan, K., et al. A Multicenter Study on the Utility of EBUS-TBNA and EUS-B-FNA in the Diagnosis of Mediastinal Lymphoma. *J Bronchology Interv Pulmonol.* 2019;26(3):199-209.

[40] Medenica, M., Bailey, S., Elkhalifa, S., Rana, D., Nadira, N. Utility of conjoined EBUS-TBNA, ROSE (rapid-on site evaluation) and flow cytometry in diagnosis of lymphoma. *European Respiratory Journal.* 2017;50(suppl 61):PA1584.

[41] Juanpere, S., Cañete, N., Ortuño, P., Martínez, S., Sanchez, G., Bernado, L. A diagnostic approach to the mediastinal masses. *Insights into imaging.* 2013;4(1):29-52.

[42] Mehta, R. M., Biraris, P., Patil, S., Singla, A., Kallur, K., Gasparini, S. Utility of EBUS-TBNA in PET-positive mediastinal lymph nodes in subjects with extra-thoracic malignancy. *PloS one.* 2019;14(3):e0213437-e0213437.

[43] Yang, B., Li, F., Shi, W., et al. Endobronchial ultrasound-guided transbronchial needle biopsy for the diagnosis of intrathoracic lymph node metastases from extrathoracic malignancies: a meta-analysis and systematic review. *Respirology.* 2014;19(6):834-841.

[44] Guarize, J., Casiraghi, M., Donghi, S., et al. EBUS-TBNA in PET-positive lymphadenopathies in treated cancer patients. *ERJ open research.* 2017;3(4):00009-02017.

[45] Nin, C. S., de Souza, V. V., do Amaral, R. H., et al. Thoracic lymphadenopathy in benign diseases: A state of the art review. *Respir Med.* 2016;112:10-17.

[46] Erbay, M., Ozsu, S., Ayaydin Murtezaoglu, E. S., et al. [Causes of mediastinal/hilar granulomatous lymphadenitis]. *Tuberk Toraks.* 2018;66(3):212-216.

[47] Statement on sarcoidosis. Joint Statement of the American Thoracic Society (ATS), the European Respiratory Society (ERS) and the World Association of Sarcoidosis and Other Granulomatous Disorders (WASOG) adopted by the ATS Board of Directors and by the ERS Executive Committee, February 1999. *Am J Respir Crit Care Med.* 1999;160(2):736-755.

[48] Goyal, A., Gupta, D., Agarwal, R., Bal, A., Nijhawan, R., Aggarwal, A. N. Value of different bronchoscopic sampling techniques in diagnosis of sarcoidosis: a prospective study of 151 patients. *J Bronchology Interv Pulmonol.* 2014;21(3):220-226.

[49] Sun, J., Yang, H., Teng, J., et al. Determining factors in diagnosing pulmonary sarcoidosis by endobronchial ultrasound-guided transbronchial needle aspiration. *Ann Thorac Surg.* 2015;99(2):441-445.

[50] Nachiappan, A. C., Rahbar, K., Shi, X., et al. Pulmonary Tuberculosis: Role of Radiology in Diagnosis and Management. *Radiographics.* 2017;37(1):52-72.

[51] Ohshimo, S., Guzman, J., Costabel, U., Bonella, F. Differential diagnosis of granulomatous lung disease: clues and pitfalls: Number 4 in the Series "Pathology for the clinician" Edited by Peter Dorfmuller and Alberto Cavazza. *Eur Respir Rev.* 2017;26(145).

[52] Madan, K., Mohan, A., Ayub, II, et al. Initial experience with endobronchial ultrasound-guided transbronchial needle aspiration (EBUS-TBNA) from a tuberculosis endemic population. *J Bronchology Interv Pulmonol.* 2014;21(3):208-214.

[53] Eom, J. S., Mok, J. H., Lee, M. K., et al. Efficacy of TB-PCR using EBUS-TBNA samples in patients with intrathoracic granulomatous lymphadenopathy. *BMC pulmonary medicine.* 2015;15:166-166.

[54] Berger, J., Zamora, F., Podgaetz, E., Andrade, R., Dincer, H. E. Usefulness of lymphoid granulomatous inflammation culture obtained by endobronchial ultrasound-guided transbronchial needle aspiration in a fungal endemic area. *Endoscopic ultrasound.* 2016;5(4):243-247.

[55] Egressy, K., Mohammed, M., Ferguson, J. S. The Use of Endobronchial Ultrasound in the Diagnosis of Subacute Pulmonary Histoplasmosis. *Diagn Ther Endosc.* 2015;2015:510863.

[56] Shah, R. A., Vempilly, J. J., Noor Ul Husnain S. M., Hegde P. Combined Endosonography Reduces Time to Diagnose Pulmonary Coccidioidomycosis. *J Bronchology Interv Pulmonol.* 2018;25(2):152-155.

In: Thoracic Lymphadenopathy
Editor: Vikas Pathak

ISBN: 978-1-53616-700-9
© 2020 Nova Science Publishers, Inc.

Chapter 10

MEDIASTINOSCOPY FOR THE DIAGNOSIS OF MEDIASTINAL AND HILAR LYMPHADENOPATHY

Mary K. Bryant[1], MD and Trevor C. Upham[2], MD
[1]University of North Carolina School of Medicine,
Chapel Hill, North Carolina, US
[2]WakeMed Health and Hospitals, Raleigh, North Carolina, US

INTRODUCTION

Mediastinal and/or hilar lymphadenopathy represent a common referral reason to pulmonary and thoracic physicians as the differential diagnosis spans benign, malignant, and infectious etiologies. While lymphadenopathy is often a surrogate of systemic disease, isolated mediastinal and/or hilar lymphadenopathy (IMHL) may be a nonspecific radiographic anomaly, reactive nodes, or a marker of a pathological disorder. Mediastinal staging techniques range from noninvasive imaging studies to a maximally invasive radical lymphadenectomy. Relying on radiographic evidence from computed tomography (CT) or positive emission tomography (PET) scans for diagnosis has been shown to be faulty and unreliable, specifically in cases of malignancy [1-3]. Surveillance of enlarged lymph nodes is rarely appropriate; therefore, sampling of nodes is recommended. Initially, a less invasive needle technique, including endobronchial ultrasound with needle aspiration (EBUS-NA), endoscopic ultrasound with needle aspiration (EUS-NA), trans-thoracic needle aspiration (TTNA), or trans-bronchial needle aspiration (TBNA) may be pursued for tissue confirmation. Many circumstances including location of the enlarged lymph node, need for significant amounts of tissue, or presumed etiology may preclude a needle technique. Additionally, similar to many other locations of lymphadenopathy, guidelines often recommend further tissue sampling after a negative or inconclusive needle technique [4].

Despite advances in imaging-guided biopsy techniques, mediastinoscopy remains the gold standard for evaluation of mediastinal lymphadenopathy since its inception over six decades ago. With a wide range of exploration potential, mediastinoscopy can be used for the histological diagnosis of tumors, infection, cysts, and inflammation. In the context of lung cancer, an accurate staging mediastinoscopy is paramount to determining the treatment and surgical plan for patients [4]. Since introduction of the videoscope in mediastinoscopy procedures by Lerut in 1989 [5], improved visualization and safety have resulted in more complete and sensitive sampling and greater teaching potential [6]. The videoscope has further allowed for the development of procedures beyond a biopsy such as video-assisted mediastinal lymphadenectomy (VAMLA) [7] and transcervical extended mediastinal lymphadenectomy (TEMLA) [8].

This chapter summarizes the role and technical considerations of mediastinoscopy as a staging and diagnostic tool for mediastinal and hilar lymphadenopathy.

INDICATIONS

While lung cancer staging, specifically for non-small cell lung cancer (NSCLC), is the most common indication for mediastinoscopy, it can also be useful in etiologies where the lymph node architecture is crucial to diagnosis, such as lymphoma [9], or the diagnosis requires more tissue than a small needle biopsy, as in sarcoidosi s [10]. Secondary causes of lymphadenopathy, often seen with IMHL, can be investigated with EBUS-TBNA. However, despite the high sensitivity of 92% previously demonstrated in the REMEDY trial with EBUS-TBNA, a negative predictive value (NPV) of 40% led to the recommendation of mediastinoscopy after negative EBUS-TBNA [11]. The differential diagnosis of secondary lymphadenopathy includes lymphoproliferative disorders [12-14], benign granulomatous disorders [15], and reactive nodes. As a diagnosis of exclusion, reactive nodes have been associated with chronic conditions such as heart failure [16], connective tissue disease [17], chronic obstructive pulmonary disease [18], and interstitial lung disease [19, 20], which can all lead to mediastinal lymphadenopathy.

For malignancy, mediastinal lymph node status (N status) is the strongest prognostic indicator of locally advanced disease [21-23]. The American College of Chest Physicians (ACCP) recommends a needle technique as the first biopsy method, but if negative, mediastinoscopy should be employed in the absence of metastatic disease [4]. The exceptions to invasive biopsy are extensive mediastinal infiltration and stage 1A tumors without suspicion of mediastinal involvement on PET or CT imaging [4]. Specific indications for mediastinoscopy according to ACCP in the case of suspected malignancy are as follows:

1) Discrete enlarged mediastinal lymph node whether or not PET-avid
2) PET-avid nodes or abnormal appearing lymph nodes on CT
3) Suspected N2 or N3 disease due to enlarged node or PET-avid node
4) Central tumor or N1 disease with a suspicion of N2 or N3 disease by imaging

The European Society of Thoracic Surgeons (ESTS) have similar guidelines for cancer staging of the mediastinum; recommended indications for pursuing invasive staging include if the needle biopsy is negative and if nodes are abnormal or enlarged, PET-avid, presumed N1 disease, or if the primary tumor is centrally located or has low PET uptake [24]. Other malignant indications for mediastinoscopy comprise of mesothelioma patients to determine surgical candidates [25], concern for lymphoma [9], mediastinal infiltration to determine histologic characteristics for treatment, and metastatic extra-thoracic malignancy who may be metastasectomy candidates [26].

CONTRAINDICATIONS

As mediastinoscopy is a relatively minimally invasive procedure, few contraindications exist. Aortic arch aneurysms are an absolute contraindication to cervical mediastinoscopy due to compression of the aorta during the procedure. Otherwise, relative contraindications include limited neck mobility for proper positioning such as with kyphosis or cervical fusion and severe atherosclerotic disease of the aortic arch, right innominate, and/or vertebral arteries. Literature has shown mediastinoscopy can be performed safely in situations previously contraindicated: history of total laryngectomy [27], existing or prior tracheostomy [27], or superior vena cava obstruction [28]. These complex cases involving patients with the before-mentioned conditions along with history of cervical or thoracic radiation, prior mediastinoscopy, or large thyroid masses should be referred to an experienced thoracic surgeon.

ROLE OF IMAGING AND PREOPERATIVE PLANNING

Imaging usually facilitates the discovery of mediastinal lymphadenopathy. Patients will present for biopsy with various imaging modalities for review and preoperative planning, and imaging should be sufficient to survey for distant metastatic disease prior to pursuing mediastinoscopy. While a chest radiograph may detect mediastinal lymphadenopathy, CT scans are the most widely used and available imaging modality for evaluation of mediastinal lymphadenopathy. An accepted definition of an enlarged mediastinal lymph node is >1 cm short-axis diameter on a transverse CT scan image [29]. In a systematic review conducted by Duke University, CT scans had a sensitivity and specificity of 51% (95% confidence interval [CI], 47-54%) and 86% (95% CI, 84-88%), respectively, for the detection of mediastinal lymphadenopathy metastasis in cases of lung cancer [29]. The low sensitivity of CT scanning results in both overstaging and understaging. However, the superior anatomic resolution of CT scanning assists in deciding which individual nodes or levels to sample and which technical approach is appropriate.

Alternatively, PET scans, an imaging modality based on the increased cellular glucose uptake of neoplastic cells, provide more sensitivity in differentiating malignant from non-malignant nodes. The pooled estimates of sensitivity and specificity for mediastinal node metastasis were 74% (95% CI, 69-79%) and 85% (95% CI, 82-88%), respectively, in a systematic review [29]. False positive PET-avid nodes can be seen in non-neoplastic conditions, such as tuberculosis or autoimmune conditions, which limit the specificity of PET scans. Per the ACCP guidelines for lung cancer, PET scans are the most accurate imaging study for non-invasive investigation of the mediastinum [29]. Combined PET-CT scans combat the limited anatomic resolution of the PET scan, so providers can discriminate individual nodes, rather than just a lymph node station. In any case, PET and CT scans should not be used alone without confirmation of suspected metastases through invasive biopsy. Evidence for this was substantiated in the Z0050 trial in 2003, showing the combination of PET and CT scans correctly identified only 53% of N2 or N3 disease [3].

Aside from imaging, a thorough history and physical exam should address and reveal any contraindications to pursuing mediastinoscopy. As a safe procedure in the ambulatory setting, mediastinoscopy does not require extensive cardiac or pulmonary clearance. However, patients must be able to tolerate general anesthesia with general endotracheal intubation or laryngeal mask airway. Anticoagulation medications and abnormal coagulation labs must be addressed preoperatively. For patients on anticoagulation, low-molecular-weight heparin can be used as a bridging therapy at least 3-5 days prior to surgery. For patients on antiplatelet therapy, low dose aspirin may be continued; however, holding high dose aspirin and/or clopidogrel should be considered in the 5-7 days preceding surgery [30].

TECHNICAL APPROACHES AND CONSIDERATIONS

Accurate assessment of the mediastinum by mediastinoscopy is critical to choosing the appropriate treatment strategy. The thoroughness of the procedure will depend on its indication. While systematic sampling should be performed for lung cancer staging, selective sampling is an appropriate strategy for presumed etiologies other than lung cancer. With selective sampling, abnormal or enlarged mediastinal or hilar lymph nodes may be targeted during mediastinoscopy for biopsy using radiographic findings on CT and PET scans.

For systematic sampling, the ACCP and ESTS both recommend biopsy of five mediastinal node stations for a complete staging procedure; these include right and left superior and inferior paratracheal nodes (stations 2L, 2R, 4L, 4R) and subcarinal nodes (station 7) [4, 31]. Ideally, assessment of a node station includes either biopsy of at least one node or a thorough exploration of that station revealing no representative nodes. Mediastinoscopy also provides access to pretracheal nodes (station 1 and 3). For those with advanced training, extended cervical mediastinoscopy can be used to evaluate lymph nodes in the subaortic (station 5) and para-aortic space (station 6). Improved visualization with a videomediastinoscope allows for complete sampling of station 7, both anterior and posterior subcarinal nodes [32]. Nodes beyond the scope of standard mediastinoscopy are inferior mediastinal nodes (station 8 and 9), aortopulmonary window nodes (station 5), and anterior mediastinal nodes (station 6). A description of the technical approaches for mediastinoscopy are discussed below in the context of staging for malignancy.

STANDARD CERVICAL

The classically described standard cervical mediastinoscopy is generally an outpatient procedure. Necessary equipment and instruments have been detailed previously [33, 34]. After general anesthesia with orotracheal intubation and hyperextension of the neck in the supine decubitus position, a transverse incision is made 1.5 fingerbreaths above the sternal notch. Midline dissection through the soft tissue and platysma will reveal the strap muscles deeply. Vertical dissection ensures avoidance of the anterior jugular veins. Care must be taken to also avoid the thyroid isthmus, which should be superior to the dissection field. Dissection should proceed deeply until the pretracheal fascia is reached. Under direct vision, the pretracheal fascia is incised sharply and lifted off the trachea with a right-angle retractor. This tissue plane should ideally be carried caudally below the level of the innominate artery. Once visualization of this plane is no longer possible, blunt digital dissection is carried out only directly over the trachea into the subcarinal space, with careful identification of the pulsation of the innominate artery and ascending aorta. This dissection plane will follow the path to the carina, often along the length of both main bronchi, and will serve as the tract for the mediastinoscope. The azygos vein, located at the tracheobronchial angle on the right, serves as an important landmark for station 4R and 10R. On the right, hilar nodes are defined those caudal to the azygos vein; while, on the left, hilar nodes are those caudal to the left pulmonary vein [35]. Once lymph node stations have been identified, blunt dissection should separate surrounding tissues to prevent injury to vascular structures. Due to the dark blue or black appearance of mediastinal lymph nodes, veins can be commonly mistaken for lymph nodes. When the tissue character is in question, the structure should be aspirated first before biopsy. After biopsy of the node with biopsy forceps, the tissue should be removed along the path of the mediastinoscope to prevent tumor implants. Hemostasis can be augmented with simple packing or hemostatic products. The wound is closed in layers with absorbable suture. Drains are not routinely used.

Without an established standardized manner of sampling, each operating surgeon should adhere to a systematic method to ensure a comprehensive staging mediastinoscopy is performed. This has been shown to correlate with more accurate staging over a selective sampling technique [36]. Additionally, a standardized method should be employed to keep track of the biopsy specimens by nodal station.

EXTENDED CERVICAL

Historically, left lung cancers required a combination of the standard cervical mediastinoscopy and Chamberlain's procedure, or left anterior mediastinoscopy, for adequate staging. Because the standard cervical mediastinoscopy is unable to sample the subaortic (station 5) and para-aortic (station 6) nodes, an extended cervical mediastinoscopy was developed as a diagnostic tool for these node levels utilizing the standard cervical mediastinoscopy incision [37-39]. Anterior mediastinal masses may also be biopsied using this technique. Popularized by Ginsberg in the late 1980s for staging left-sided bronchogenic carcinoma, the extended cervical approach follows a standard mediastinoscopy in terms of preoperative assessment, contraindications, required anesthesia, and patient positioning. The same instruments required for a standard procedure may be used for the extended approach. Incision and soft tissue dissection is performed as described above for a standard cervical mediastinoscopy. Once the dissection reaches the innominate artery, a plane is developed over or under the left innominate vein and the aorta. A mediastinoscope can then be advanced over the aortic arch to reach station 5 and 6 nodes, between the innominate artery and left carotid artery. This technique can be slightly modified as an alternative to minimally invasive methods for diagnosis of a pre-aortic mass, where a retrosternal plane is developed to access the origin of the innominate artery for biopsy of an anterior mediastinal mass.

REMEDIASTINOSCOPY

Initially considered a contraindication to mediastinoscopy, prior mediastinoscopy has been demonstrated to be safe and instrumental in preventing unnecessary thoracotomies [40-42]. Indications include initial sampling error, restaging after induction therapy, mediastinitis and other inflammatory conditions, recurrent malignancy, and second primary lung cancer. After reincising the prior cervical incision, sharp dissection should proceed through the dense adhesions to reach the pretracheal space. To avoid injury to the usually scarred brachiocephalic trunk, a left paratracheal approach has been described where a tunnel for the mediastinoscope is developed to the level of the aorta [43]. From this location, the trachea can be crossed to biopsy the right paratracheal nodes (4R). While staying posterior to the right pulmonary artery, station 7 can be reached by following this pretracheal plane. Deep to the aortic arch fascia, the former station 3 nodes are now 4R and 2R.

For restaging procedures, comparison of the same stations is important to determine response to induction therapy. In the case of locally advanced stage III NSCLC, potential mediastinal downstaging may allow for surgical resection, whereas persistent or progressive disease will not benefit from resection [44].

VEMLA AND VAMLA

Newer techniques have expanded the use of mediastinoscopy from a diagnostic procedure to a therapeutic procedure. A core principle of oncological surgery is removal of the complete draining lymphatic system along with the primary tumor for surgically curable malignancies. Depending on the laterality of the primary tumor, concurrent lymphadenectomy and primary lesion resection can prove to be difficult, time-intensive, and invasive. Further, with complete lymphadenectomy, mediastinal staging is more accurate than conventional mediastinoscopy.

Although long-term data is lacking, VAMLA and VEMLA have been increasingly used for staging and definitive treatment of the mediastinum.

First described by Hürtgen in 2002, VAMLA was made possible through the development of the Linder- Hürtgen mediastinoscope with bimanual spreadable blades [7]. Aside from avoiding repeat mediastinoscopy after neoadjuvant therapy, VAMLA unifies multiple procedures by combining staging and treatment, such as VAMLA plus extended mediastinoscopy for left-sided tumors, mediastinoscopic ultrasound, or video-assisted thoracoscopic surgery (VATS) lobectomy. Field radiation and radiofrequency ablation have also been performed in conjunction with VAMLA. Similar to conventional mediastinoscopy, the targeted lymph nodes of VAMLA are stations 2, 4, and 7 bilaterally. However, the procedure can be tailored to address stations 1, 3a, 8, 10, and 11R if a videomediastinoscope is used, and station 5 and 6L, if an extended mediastinoscopy approach is taken. Technical details of VAMLA have been outlined by Witte et al. [8]. Case series of VAMLA have shown a similar lymph node yield as open mediastinal dissection [7] with a relatively low complication rate [45].

VEMLA expanded upon VAMLA to include components of the extended cervical mediastinoscopy to remove stations not accessible by VAMLA. Operating through a cervical collar incision, stations 1, 2R, 2L, 3a, 4R, 4L, 5, 6, 7, and 8 can be completely removed with the aid of a videomediastinoscope. This technique mirrors the completeness of the Hata et al. superradical bilateral mediastinal dissection, with the exception of station 9 [46]. Mobilization the great vessels of the neck and elevation of the sternum provides the superior exposure of the mediastinum for this procedure without the need for bilateral thoracotomy or sternotomy. Current data suggest the number of lymph nodes removed with TEMLA is superior to that of thoracotomy and VATS lymphadenectomy [47]. Drawbacks of this procedure include the long operative times and subsequent scarring of the mediastinum, complicating future lung resections if not performed in the early postoperative period.

PITFALLS AND COMPLICATIONS

Mediastinoscopy has remained the gold standard of mediastinal biopsy because of its accuracy in determining nodal status and pathologic etiologies of mediastinal lymphadenopathy. However, this has been threatened by reports of inadequate lymph node sampling and no widely accepted standardization of the procedure. In a commonly cited study, Little et. al reported that fewer than 50% of mediastinoscopies performed by general surgeons yielded any lymph node tissue [48]. To the contrary, in a single center case series of thoracic surgeon-performed mediastinoscopies, lymph node tissue was obtained 100% of the time [49]. EBUS-FNA has been touted as an equivalent alternative to mediastinoscopy [50] and precedes mediastinoscopy in the ACCP guidelines as the recommended initial staging procedure [29]. Opposing research has demonstrated the higher false negative rate of these minimally invasive needle techniques versus mediastinoscopy. Using pooled data, the overall false negative rates were 16% for EUS-NA and 24% for EBUS-FNA [51]. For comparison, false negative rates of video mediastinoscopy are reported around 7% [4]. Despite the imperative nature of mediastinoscopy in lung cancer staging, it remains standard of care to follow this initial sampling with further biopsy and lymphadenectomy during the primary lung resection.

While mediastinoscopy has reported low morbidity and mortality, clinicians should be aware of potential complications in order to educate patients preoperatively about the risks of each technique. For conventional mediastinoscopy, the complication rate is approximately 3% across series, with major complications less than 1% and mortality below 0.5% [52, 53]. In a single center case series, unexpected hospital admission or readmission rates were approximately 0.5% [49].

For procedure related complications, injury to vital surrounding structures including the esophagus, recurrent laryngeal nerve (RLN), pleura, and great vessels are rare, but can result in significant morbidity and possible sternotomy or thoracotomy. Electrocautery should be used with caution to prevent several of these complications. The risk of RLN injury can be minimized with judicious use of electrocautery in the left paratracheal and tracheobronchial angle areas. The risk of esophageal perforation decreases with avoiding electrocautery in the subcarinal space. While violation of the pleural space is uncommon and routine postoperative x-rays are not indicated, care must be taken in the right paratracheal area, especially with emphysematous lungs, as this is a common entry point into the pleural cavity. Mechanical ventilation during the procedure may also rupture existing blebs or bullae leading to pneumothorax. Because bleeding is commonly encountered and can lead to a mediastinal hematoma if proper hemostasis is not obtained prior to closure, use of electrocautery can be beneficial along with temporarily packing biopsied areas and use of absorbable hemostatic agents in the field. Other reported complications include cervical wound infection, mediastinitis, ventricular fibrillation, cerebrovascular accident, tracheobronchial injury, chylomediastinum, incisional metastasis, and intraoperative death.

Patients should be counseled preoperatively that catastrophic bleeding would necessitate a sternotomy to repair a bleeding vessel. In cases of azygous injury with planned subsequent right sided surgery, a right thoracotomy can be considered.

Conclusion

In determining the pathology of mediastinal and hilar lymphadenopathy, mediastinoscopy provides an efficient, accurate, and safe approach to biopsy. Integration of imaging findings with pathologic results from mediastinoscopy prevents most patients with mediastinal lymph node metastasis from undergoing non-curative surgical resection. Beyond diagnosis and staging, the technical variants of mediastinoscopy, including the therapeutic VAMLA and VEMLA, have transformed this procedure into an even more important tool as a treatment modality for the mediastinum. In summary, while more minimally invasive techniques have attempted to surpass mediastinoscopy, data and long-term outcomes support the utility of mediastinoscopy as the gold standard mechanism for accurate lung cancer staging and histologic evaluation of the mediastinum.

REFERENCES

[1] Antoch G., Saoudi N., Kuchl H., Al E. Accuracy of whole-body dual-modality fluorine-18-2-fluoro-2-deoxy-D-glucose positron emission tomography and computed tomography (FDG-PET/CT) for tumor staging in solid tumors: comparison with CT and PET. *J Clin Oncol.* 2004;22(21):4357-4368.

[2] Lardinois D., Weder W., Hany T., Al E. Staging of non-small-cell lung cancer with integrated positron-emission tomography and computed tomography. *N Eng J Med.* 2003;348(25):2500-2507.

[3] Reed C. E., Harpole D., Posther K., et al. Results of the American College of Surgeons Oncology Group Z0050 trial: the utility of positron emission tomography in staging potentially operable non-small cell lung cancer. *J Thorac Cardiovasc Surg.* 2003;126(6):1943-1951.

[4] Silvestri G. A., Gonzalez A. V., Jantz MA, et al. Methods for staging non-small cell lung cancer: Diagnosis and management of lung cancer, 3rd ed: American college of chest physicians evidence-based clinical practice guidelines. *Chest.* 2013;143(5 SUPPL):e211S-e250S.

[5] Coosemans, W., Lerut, T., Van Raemdonck, D. Thoracoscopic surgery: the Belgian experience. *Ann Thorc Surg.* 1993;56:721-730.

[6] Adebibe, M., Jarral, O. A., Shipolini, A. R., McCormack, D. J. Does video-assisted mediastinoscopy have a better lymph node yield and safety profile than conventional mediastinoscopy? *Interact Cardiovasc Thorac Surg.* 2012;14(3):316-319.

[7] Hürtgen, M., Friedel, G., Toomes, H., Fritz, P. Radical video-assisted mediastinoscopic lymphadenectomy (VAMLA)--technique and first results. *Eur J Cardiothorac Surg.* 2002;21:348-351.

[8] Kuzdzał, J., Zieliński, M., Papla, B., et al. Transcervical extended mediastinal lymphadenectomy - The new operative technique and early results in lung cancer staging. *Eur J Cardio-thoracic Surg.* 2005;27(3):384-390.

[9] Vitolo, U., Seymour, J., Martelli, M., et al. Extranodal diffuse large B-cell lymphoma (DLBCL) and primary mediastinal B-cell lymphoma:

ESMO Clinical Practice Guidelines for diagnosis, treatment and follow-up. *Ann Oncol.* 2016;27(suppl 5):v91-v102.

[10] Govender P, Berman J. The diagnosis of sarcoidosis. *Clin Chest Med.* 2015;36(4):585-602.

[11] Navani, N., Lawrence, D., Kolvekar, S., Al, E. Endobronchial ultrasound-guided transbronchial needle aspiration prevents mediastinoscopies in the diagnosis of isolated mediastinal lymphadenopathy: a prospective trial. *Am J Crit Care.* 2012;186:255-260.

[12] Talat, N., Schulte, K. Castleman's disease: systematic analysis of 416 patients from the literature. *Oncologist.* 2011;16:1316-1324.

[13] Curtin, J. J., Murray, J., LA, A., Al, E. Mediastinal lymph node enlargement and splenomegaly in primary hypogammaglobulinaemia. *Clin Radiol.* 1995;50:489-491.

[14] Wheat, L. J., Conces, D., Allen, S., Al, E. Pulmonary histoplasmosis syndromes: recognition, diagnosis, and management. *Semin Respir Crit Care Med.* 2004;25:129-144.

[15] Garwood, S., Judson, M., G. S., Al, E. Endobronchial ultrasound for the diagnosis of pulmonary sarcoidosis. *Chest.* 2007;132:1298-1304.

[16] Chabbert, V., Canevet G, Baixas C, Al E. Mediastinal lymphadenopathy in congestive heart failure: a sequential CT evaluation with clinical and echocardiographic correlations. *Eur Radiol.* 2004;14:881-889.

[17] Martinez, F. J., Karlinsky, J., Gale, M., Al, E. Intrathoracic lymphadenopathy. A rare manifestation of rheumatoid pulmonary disease. *Chest.* 1990;97:1010-1012.

[18] Kirchner, J., Kirchner, E., Goltz, J., Al, E. Enlarged hilar and mediastinal lymph nodes in chronic obstructive pulmonary disease. *J Med Imaging Radiat Oncol.* 2010;54:333-338.

[19] Bergin, C., Castellino, R. Mediastinal lymph node enlargement on CT scans in patients with usual interstitial pneumonitis. *AJR Am J Roentgenol.* 1990;154:251-254.

[20] Souza, C. A., Muller, N., Lee, K., Al, E. Idiopathic interstitial pneumonias: prevalence of mediastinal lymph node enlargement in 206 patients. *AJR Am J Roentgenol.* 2006;186:995-999.

[21] Vallières, E., Shepherd, F., Crowley, J., et al. The IASLC Lung Cancer Staging Project: proposals regarding the relevance of TNM in the pathologic staging of small cell lung cancer in the forthcoming (seventh) edition of the TNM classification for lung cancer. *J Thorc Oncol.* 2009;4:1049-1059.

[22] Howington, J. A., Blum, M., Chang, A., Balekian, A., Murthy, S. Treatment of stage I and II non-small cell lung cancer: Diagnosis and management of lung cancer, 3rd ed: American College of Chest Physicians evidence-based clinical practice guidelines. *Chest.* 2013;143(5 suppl):e278S-e313S.

[23] Asamura, H., Chansky, K., Crowley, J., et al. The International Association for the Study of Lung Cancer Lung Cancer Staging Project: Proposals for the Revision of the N Descriptors in the Forthcoming 8th Edition of the TNM Classification for Lung Cancer. *J Thorc Oncol.* 2015;10:1675-1684.

[24] De Leyn, P., Lardinois, D., Van Schil PE, et al. ESTS guidelines for preoperative lymph node staging for non-small cell lung cancer. *Eur J Cardio-thoracic Surg.* 2007;32(1):1-8.

[25] Stahel, R., Weder, W., Lievans, Y., E F. Malignant pleural mesothelioma: ESMO Clinical Practice Guidelines for diagnosis, treatment and follow-up. *Ann Oncol.* 2010;21(Supplement 5):v126-v128.

[26] Riquet, M., Berna, P., Brian, E., et al. Intrathoracic lymph node metastases from extrathoracic carcinoma: the place for surgery. *Ann Thorc Surg.* 2009;88:200-205.

[27] Yamada, K., Kumar, P., Goldstraw, P. Cervical mediastinoscopy after total laryngectomy and radiotherapy: its feasibility. *Eur J Cardiothorac Surg.* 2002;21:71-73.

[28] Dosios, T., Theakos, N., Chatziantoniou, C. Cervical mediastinoscopy and anterior mediastinotomy in superior vena cava obstruction. *Chest.* 2005;128:1551-1556.

[29] Silvestri, G. A., Gould, M. K., Margolis, M. L., Al E. Noninvasive staging of non-small cell lung cancer: ACCP evidenced-based clinical practice guidelines (2nd edition). *Chest*. 2007;132(3 suppl):178S-201S. doi:10.1378/chest.07-1360.

[30] Douketis, J. D., Berger, P., Dunn, A., et al. The perioperative management of antithrombotic therapy: American College of Chest Physicians Evidence-Based Clinical Practice Guidelines (8th Edition). *Chest*. 2008;133(6 suppl):299S-339S.

[31] Schil, P. V., Dooms, C., Lardinois, D., et al. Revised ESTS guidelines for preoperative mediastinal lymph node staging for non-small-cell lung cancer. *Eur J Cardio-Thoracic Surg*. 2014;45(5):787-798.

[32] Sayar, A., Citak, N., Metin, M., et al. Comparison of video-assisted mediastinoscopy and video-assisted mediastinoscopic lymphadenectomy for lung cancer. *Gen Thorac Cardiovasc Surg*. 2011;59:793-798.

[33] Rami-Porta, R., Call, S., Serra-Mitjans, M. Mediastinoscopy. In: *The Transcervical Approach in Thoracic Surgery*.; 2014:9-27.

[34] Wilson, J. L., Vallières, E. Mediastinoscopy and mediastinotomy. In: *Operative Thoracic Surgery, 6th Edition*. 107-116.

[35] Rusch, V. W., Asamura, H., Watanabe, H., Giroux, D., Rami-Porta, R., Goldstraw, P. The IASLC lung cancer staging project: a proposal for a new international lymph node map in the forthcoming seventh edition of the TNM classification for lung cancer. *J Thorc Oncol*. 2009;4:568-577.

[36] Detterbeck, F. C. Integration of mediastinal staging techniques for lung cancer. *Semin Thorac Cardiovasc Surg*. 2007;19(3):217-224.

[37] Hürtgen, M., Witte B. History of extended cervical mediastinoscopy. *Eur J Cardiothorac Surg*. 2009;35:745.

[38] Ginsberg, R. J., Rice, T. W., Goldberg, M., Al, E. Extended cervical mediastinoscopy. A single staging procedure for bronchogenic carcinoma of the left upper lobe. *J Thorac Cardiovasc Surg*. 1987;94:673-678.

[39] Ginsberg, R. J. Extended cervical mediastinoscopy. *Chest Surg Clin N Am*. 1996;6:21-30.

[40] Palva, T., Palva A., Karja, J. Re-mediastinoscopy. *Arch Otolaryngol.* 1975;101:748-750.

[41] Lewis, R., Sisler, G., Mackenzie, J. Repeat mediastinoscopy. *Ann Thorc Surg.* 1984;37:147-149.

[42] Van Schil, P. The restaging issue. *Lung Cancer.* 2003;42(Suppl 1):S39-45.

[43] Van Schil, P. E., De Waele, M. A second mediastinoscopy: how to decide and how to do it? *Eur J Cardiothorac Surg.* 2008;33:703-706.

[44] Albain, K. S., Swann, R., Rusch, V., Al, E. Radiotherapy plus chemotherapy with or without surgical resection for stage III non-small-cell lung cancer: a phase III randomised controlled trial. *Lancet.* 2009;374:379-386.

[45] Witte, B., Wolf, M., Hurtgen, M., Toomes, H. Video-assisted mediastinoscopic surgery: clinical feasibility and accuracy of mediastinal lymph node staging. *Ann Thorc Surg.* 2006;82:1821-1827.

[46] Hata, E., Hayakawa, K., Miyamoto, H., Hayashida, R. Rationale for extended lymphadenectomy for lung cancer. *Theor Surg.* 1990;5:19-25.

[47] Jiao, J., Magistrelli, P., Goldstraw, P. The value of cervical mediastinoscopy combined with anterior mediastinotomy in the perioperative evaluation of bronchogenic carcinoma of the left upper lobe. *Eur J Cardiothorac Surg.* 1997;11:450-454.

[48] Little, A., Rusch, V., Bonner, J., Al, E. Patterns of surgical care of lung cancer patients. *Ann Thorc Surg.* 2005;80:2051-2056.

[49] Wei, B., Bryant, A. S., Minnich, D. J., Cerfolio, R. J. The safety and efficacy of mediastinoscopy when performed by general thoracic surgeons. *Ann Thorac Surg.* 2014;97(6):1878-1884.

[50] Yasufuku, K., Pierre, A., Darling, G., Al, E. A prospective controlled trial of endobronchial ultrasound-guided transbronchial needle aspiration compared with mediastinoscopy for mediastinal lymph node staging of lung cancer. *J Thorac Cardiovasc Surg.* 2011;142(6):1393-1400.e1.

[51] Detterbeck, F., Jantz, M., Wallace, M., Al, E. Invasive mediastinal staging of lung cancer: ACCP evidence-based clinical practice guidelines (2nd edition). *Chest*. 2007;132(suppl 3):202s-220s.

[52] Hammoud, Z., Anderson, R., Meyers, B., et al. The current role of mediastinoscopy in the evaluation of thoracic diseases. *J Thorac Cardiovasc Surg*. 1999;118:894-899.

[53] Kleims, G., Savic, B. Complications of mediastinoscopy. *Endoscopy*. 1979;1:9-12.

About the Editor

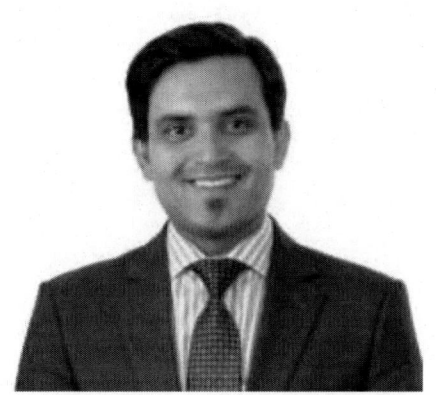

Vikas Pathak, MD, FACP, FCCP, ATSF, DAABIP
Interventional Pulmonology and Critical Care Medicine
Medical Director, Division of Pulmonary and Critical Care Medicine,
Department of Medicine, Newport News, Virginia, US
Associate Professor of Medicine, Campbell University School of Medicine
Fayetteville, North Carolina, USA

Dr. Pathak did his medical schooling from Nepal, an Asian country located in the foothills of Himalaya. He did his residency from New York and moved to University of North Carolina, Chapel Hill for his Pulmonary and Critical Care (PCCM) training. He eventually went on to do

Interventional Pulmonology fellowship at Virginia Commonwealth University, Richmond. Dr. Pathak has been very actively involved in research and has published several manuscripts in his short career. He has been actively involved in several professional societies including ATS, Chest, ERS, SCCM and AABIP. He has also received recognition through awards in his medical school (honors in Anatomy, Pathology and Surgery), residency (best resident of the year - twice) and fellowship (Philip Bromberg award for academic excellence). He is also very active in medical education and mentored several medical students and residents. He was also elected as the secretary-treasurer of North Carolina Thoracic Society. He has been practicing Interventional Pulmonology and Critical Care Medicine since he graduated from Interventional Pulmonology fellowship from Virginia Commonwealth University. He is currently serving as the medical director of the division of Pulmonary and Critical Care Medicine at Riverside Health System, Virginia.

INDEX

A

access, 40, 89, 120, 126, 129, 131, 135, 156, 158
acid, 67
acrocyanosis, 111
acute infection, 62, 63, 70
acute respiratory distress syndrome, 74
ADA, 68
adenocarcinoma, 20, 21, 38, 43
adenoma, 110
adenopathy, 38, 63, 66, 96, 120, 129, 136, 138, 139, 140, 144
adenosine, 68
adhesions, 40, 159
adrenal gland, 135
adrenal glands, 135
adult T-cell, 52
adults, 51, 78, 110
advancement, 89
aerospace, 104
African American women, 82
African Americans, 81
African-American, 81
age, 82, 83, 110, 113, 115

airways, 29, 91
alveoli, 62, 101
amyloidosis, 36, 39, 88, 140
anatomy, 24, 30, 40, 141
anemia, 111
angiography, 48
anorexia, 104
antibody, 2, 69, 70, 72, 112
anticoagulation, 155
antigen, 69, 70, 71
anti-inflammatories, 90
aorta, 30, 42, 126, 153, 157, 158, 159
apex, 5, 123
artery, 5, 126, 157, 158
aspirate, 69
aspiration, 19, 21, 22, 32, 33, 41, 46, 47, 48, 49, 55, 57, 67, 72, 89, 91, 120, 124, 126, 130, 131, 132, 134, 142, 143, 147, 150, 165, 169
assessment, 14, 18, 24, 107, 113, 155, 156, 158
asymptomatic, 14, 15, 37, 48, 64, 83
audit, 131, 144
autoimmune hemolytic anemia, 110
autopsy, 18

avoidance, 156

B

benign, xi, 32, 36, 37, 38, 39, 45, 48, 60, 61, 76, 92, 94, 106, 110, 116, 119, 130, 136, 140, 146, 149, 151
benign disease, xi, 36, 60, 92, 106, 130, 146
berylliosis, 87, 88, 89, 137
beryllium, 104, 105
bilateral, 5, 51, 53, 66, 72, 77, 83, 84, 85, 87, 88, 102, 111, 138, 160
biomarkers, 23, 112
biopsy, 19, 35, 37, 38, 41, 42, 52, 55, 56, 67, 68, 69, 72, 88, 89, 90, 95, 112, 114, 129, 130, 146, 150, 151, 152, 153, 154, 155, 157, 158, 159, 161, 163
biopsy needle, 42
bleeding, 41, 162
blindness, 83
blood, 19, 69, 71, 72, 105, 132
blood smear, 69
body fluid, 72
bone, 54, 69, 112
bone marrow, 54, 69
bone marrow biopsy, 69
brain, 24, 64
branching, 102
breast cancer, 31, 36, 45
breast carcinoma, 32
bronchiectasis, 86, 95
bronchioles, 100, 102
bronchoscopy, 49, 67, 72, 78, 129, 141
bronchus, 8, 35, 126, 127

C

calcification, 36, 61, 67, 102, 103
calcifications, 63, 88, 102
calcium, 84
CAM, 21
cancer, xi, 14, 19, 24, 25, 26, 27, 32, 33, 34, 38, 45, 94, 120, 133, 140, 142, 144, 146, 151, 152, 155, 164, 166, 168
cancer death, 24, 133, 144
cancer screening, 14
candidates, 152
capillary, 131
carbon, 99
carcinoid tumor, 18, 38
carcinoma, 14, 20, 21, 22, 33, 35, 43, 136, 158, 167, 168, 169
Caucasians, 81
CBC, 110
cell differentiation, 43
challenges, 31, 97
chemicals, 98
chemotherapy, 23, 114, 116, 117, 169
chest radiography, 83, 85, 86, 95
CHF, 87
children, vii, 62, 78
chondrosarcoma, 36
chronic obstructive pulmonary disease, 94, 99, 140, 151, 166
circulation, 18
classification, 3, 16, 18, 24, 46, 56, 57, 85, 106, 140, 141, 166, 168
clinical presentation, 14, 59, 69, 95, 101
clinical symptoms, 14
clinical trials, 73
coal, 99, 100
coal dust, 99
coccidioidomycosis, 71, 77, 88, 94, 138, 139
collagen, 90, 100, 102, 107
colon, 32
colon cancer, 32
color, iv, 130
colorectal cancer, 45
common presenting symptoms, 113
common symptoms, 14
communication, 120, 133
complement, 69, 71, 114

Index

complexity, 30
compliance, 73
complications, 41, 96, 112, 132, 161, 162
compression, 153
computed tomography, 27, 29, 48, 57, 78, 99, 150, 163, 164
congestive heart failure, 94, 165
Congress, iv
connective tissue, 29, 94, 151
consensus, 106
Consensus, 49
consolidation, 62, 63, 64, 66, 73, 87, 103, 116
control measures, 104
controversial, 23
convergence, 103, 105
COPD, 87, 99, 140
correlation, 48, 91, 96, 107, 138
cost, 97, 120
cough, 14, 15, 64, 65, 67, 83, 99, 101, 104
counseling, 55
cricoid cartilage, 4, 121
crystalline, 101, 102
CT chest, xii, 15, 16, 18, 84
CT scan, xi, 19, 28, 34, 35, 37, 39, 45, 56, 61, 62, 63, 133, 154, 166
culture, 67, 69, 71, 72, 88, 139, 147
cytokines, 101, 102
cytology, 139, 144
cytomegalovirus, 116
cytometry, 113, 136, 145
cytoplasm, 35

D

database, 16
deficiency, 110, 116
deposition, 84
dermatologist, 81
destruction, 115
detection, 14, 69, 70, 105, 133, 139, 154

diaphragm, 3, 8, 16, 29, 127
differential diagnosis, xi, 28, 29, 36, 51, 75, 110, 149, 151
discordance, 137
disease activity, 117
disease progression, 103, 105, 112
diseases, 38, 51, 84, 89, 92, 94, 95, 96, 98, 106, 109, 137, 140, 146, 170
disorder, 2, 95, 110, 115, 117, 150
distribution, 30, 39, 82, 85, 95, 100, 102
DNA, 71, 72
dosing, 90
drainage, 2, 4, 17, 29
dyspnea, 14, 15, 65, 74, 83, 99, 101, 104

E

EBUS-TBNA, xii, 33, 43, 46, 47, 55, 57, 67, 68, 90, 120, 128, 129, 131, 132, 134, 135, 136, 138, 139, 140, 141, 142, 143, 144, 145, 146, 147, 151
EBV infection, 66, 114
education, 172
effusion, 68
electrocautery, 162
ELISA, 69
emission, 150, 164
emphysema, 86, 101, 103
endoscope, 132
endotracheal intubation, 155
enlargement, 15, 19, 45, 87, 107, 111, 140, 165, 166
enzyme, 70
enzyme-linked immunoassay, 70
epidemiology, 30
episcleritis, 83
Epstein-Barr virus, 113, 114, 117
equipment, 72, 156
ERS, 106, 108, 146, 172
erythema nodosum, 64, 83
esophageal cancer, 32

esophagus, 8, 29, 30, 132, 162
etiology, 65, 94, 110, 116, 140, 150
Europe, 112
EUS, x, xii, 19, 32, 36, 40, 46, 67, 119, 120, 125, 126, 127, 128, 132, 134, 135, 139, 140, 142, 144, 145, 150, 161
evidence, 25, 37, 48, 75, 91, 106, 113, 136, 142, 150, 164, 166, 169
examinations, 97
excision, 110
exclusion, 67, 151
excretion, 84
exertion, 83, 104
exposure, 66, 82, 98, 99, 104, 160

F

false negative, 19, 161
false positive, 19
fascia, 156, 159
fat, 29, 61
fever, 64, 67, 83, 104, 111, 115
F-FDG PET, 48
fibers, 100
fibroblast proliferation, 102
fibroblasts, 90, 101, 102
fibrosis, 77, 82, 94, 96, 100, 101, 102, 103, 104, 105, 106, 107, 108, 138
fibrous cap, 102
fibrous tissue, 90, 100
fixation, 69, 71
flex, 131
fluid, 1, 13, 68, 105
fluorine, 163
formation, 61, 82, 89, 100, 102, 104
fungal infection, 61, 139
fungus, 63, 69, 72
fusion, 153

G

gallium, 54
gastric lavage, 78
gastroenterologist, 135
gastrointestinal involvement, 64
general anesthesia, 40, 129, 142, 155, 156
general surgeon, 161
genes, 82, 116
genetics, 55
genitourinary tract, 36
gland, 29
glucocorticoid, 90
glucose, 154, 163
granulomas, 85, 90, 104, 137
grouping, 2, 3, 6, 9, 122, 123
growth, 23, 37, 71, 114
growth factor, 23
guidance, 23
guidelines, xi, 25, 35, 44, 48, 106, 142, 150, 152, 154, 161, 164, 166, 167, 169

H

HCG, 45
head and neck cancer, 45
health, 79, 132
heart failure, 37, 140, 151
hemangioma, 57, 111
hematoma, 162
hemolytic anemia, 115
hemoptysis, 14, 15, 64, 115
hemostasis, 162
hepatitis, 104
hepatosplenomegaly, 64, 115
hilar lymphadenopathy, xi, xii, 14, 28, 32, 38, 39, 41, 47, 51, 53, 55, 56, 59, 62, 66, 77, 85, 105, 109, 137, 149, 151, 163
histology, 95
histoplasmosis, 62, 70, 74, 77, 88, 94, 137, 138, 139, 165

history, 16, 67, 68, 95, 99, 112, 153, 155
HIV, 78, 111, 113
HIV-1, 111
HLA, 82
hospitalization, 78, 81, 96
host, 69, 84, 114
hub, 29
human, 111
human immunodeficiency virus, 111
humidity, 82
hyaline, 90
hypercalcemia, 83, 84, 104
hypercalciuria, 84
hypergammaglobulinemia, 115
hyperplasia, 96
hypersensitivity, 87, 104, 137
hyperthyroidism, 84
hypertonic saline, 67
hypertrichosis, 111
hypoxia, 74

I

IASLC guidelines, xi
ibuprofen, 88
identification, 68, 72, 157
identity, 95
idiopathic, 94, 95, 96, 98, 106, 108, 112, 116
IFN, 82
iliac crest, 112
image, 154
images, 57
imaging modalities, 27, 99, 153
immune cells, 1, 2, 82
immune regulation, 114
immune response, 117
immunity, 77
immunocompromised, 70, 71, 72, 75, 111
immunofluorescence, 72
immunoglobulin(s), 110, 111, 113

immunoreactivity, 35
immunosuppression, 113
in vitro, 114
incidence, xi, 24, 27, 32, 73, 81, 82, 88, 104
India, 141
individuals, 66, 67, 69, 70, 71, 72, 74, 99, 111
indolent, 28, 52, 59, 112
induction, 23, 67, 69, 72, 73, 74, 158, 159
induction chemotherapy, 23
industry, 104
infection, 61, 62, 63, 64, 65, 66, 69, 70, 72, 75, 77, 78, 88, 111, 133, 139, 150
inflammation, 2, 28, 45, 62, 86, 133, 137, 147, 150
influenza, 63, 66, 75, 78
influenza virus, 63
ingestion, 98, 102
initiation, 75
injury, iv, 101, 102, 157, 159, 162, 163
innominate, 5, 7, 124, 153, 156, 158
inoculation, 70
interferon, 66, 115
interstitial lung disease, 37, 82, 94, 95, 96, 97, 107, 151
interstitial pneumonia, 94, 95, 98, 106, 107, 166
interstitial pneumonitis, 116, 166
intervention, 100
intraocular, 83
intraocular pressure, 83
ipsilateral, 4, 18, 128
irradiation, 24
isolation, 67
isoniazid, 64, 73, 74, 78, 79, 87
issues, 90

K

kill, 62
kyphosis, 153

L

laboratory studies, 110
laryngeal cancer, 32
laryngectomy, 153, 167
latency, 101
laterality, 10, 159
Latin America, 108
lead, 38, 61, 62, 84, 86, 88, 102, 113, 116, 151, 162
left atrium, 126
leprosy, 89
lesions, 29, 37, 45, 54, 100, 104, 105, 112
leukopenia, 115
ligament, 7, 8, 127
ligand, 23
lipoma, 136
liver, 18, 110, 112, 120, 135
liver failure, 112
lobectomy, 23, 160
localization, 128, 130
Louisiana, 13
low dose CT scan, xi
lower respiratory tract infection, 63
lung cancer, xi, 2, 3, 14, 15, 18, 19, 24, 25, 30, 33, 34, 36, 39, 41, 43, 45, 46, 48, 76, 84, 88, 89, 94, 120, 129, 133, 134, 136, 140, 141, 142, 144, 145, 150, 151, 154, 155, 158, 159, 161, 163, 164, 166, 167, 168, 169
lung cancer screening, xi, 14, 15
lung disease, 90, 94, 95, 96, 97, 98, 105, 107, 108, 147
lung function, 91, 96
lung transplantation, 77
lupus, 83
lying, 10
lymph, xi, xii, 1, 2, 3, 4, 5, 6, 7, 8, 9, 10, 14, 15, 16, 17, 18, 19, 22, 23, 24, 27, 28, 29, 30, 31, 32, 33, 35, 36, 37, 38, 39, 40, 42, 43, 45, 46, 47, 48, 49, 51, 52, 53, 54, 55, 56, 57, 59, 60, 61, 62, 63, 64, 65, 66, 67, 69, 72, 75, 76, 77, 83, 84, 85, 87, 88, 89, 90, 92, 93, 94, 95, 96, 97, 101, 102, 105, 106, 107, 109, 110, 111, 115, 116, 118, 119, 120, 121, 122, 123, 124, 125, 126, 127, 128, 129, 130, 131, 133, 134, 135, 136, 137, 139, 140, 141, 145, 146, 147, 149, 150, 151, 152, 153, 154, 155, 156, 157, 160, 161, 163, 164, 165, 166, 167, 168, 169
lymph node, xi, 1, 2, 3, 4, 5, 6, 7, 8, 9, 10, 14, 15, 16, 17, 18, 19, 22, 23, 24, 27, 29, 30, 31, 32, 34, 35, 36, 37, 38, 40, 42, 45, 46, 47, 48, 53, 54, 56, 57, 60, 61, 62, 75, 76, 77, 87, 89, 90, 93, 96, 97, 102, 103, 105, 107, 110, 111, 116, 120, 121, 122, 123, 124, 125, 126, 127, 128, 129, 130, 131, 133, 134, 135, 136, 137, 139, 140, 141, 145, 146, 150, 151, 152, 154, 155, 156, 157, 160, 161, 163, 164, 165, 166, 167, 168, 169
lymph node stations, xi, 3, 4, 6, 9, 41, 120, 122, 123, 134, 157
lymph nodes, 1, 2, 3, 4, 5, 6, 7, 8, 10, 14, 16, 17, 18, 19, 23, 24, 27, 29, 30, 32, 34, 35, 36, 37, 38, 40, 45, 48, 54, 57, 61, 62, 75, 76, 77, 87, 89, 93, 96, 97, 102, 103, 105, 110, 111, 116, 120, 121, 124, 125, 126, 127, 128, 129, 130, 131, 133, 134, 135, 136, 137, 140, 145, 150, 152, 155, 156, 157, 160, 166
lymphadenitis, 146
lymphadenopathy, xi, xii, 2, 14, 16, 19, 27, 28, 30, 31, 32, 33, 36, 37, 38, 39, 41, 43, 47, 49, 51, 52, 53, 55, 56, 57, 59, 60, 61, 62, 63, 64, 65, 66, 67, 69, 72, 77, 83, 85, 87, 88, 92, 93, 94, 95, 96, 97, 101, 102, 105, 106, 107, 109, 111, 115, 116, 118, 119, 133, 137, 141, 146, 147, 149, 150, 151, 153, 161, 163, 165
lymphatic fluid, 1
lymphatic network, xi

lymphatic system, 2, 13, 159
lymphatic vessels, 1
lymphocytes, 2, 90, 132
lymphoid, 1, 96, 130, 147
lymphoid tissue, 130
lymphoma, 2, 23, 52, 53, 54, 55, 56, 57, 58, 87, 88, 94, 110, 113, 114, 115, 116, 136, 145, 151, 152, 164

M

macrophages, 62, 82, 84, 100, 101, 102, 104
magnetic resonance, 56
magnetic resonance imaging, 56
majority, 64
malignancy, 29, 30, 32, 33, 35, 37, 40, 45, 46, 47, 49, 53, 87, 114, 136, 146, 150, 152, 153, 156, 159
malignant melanoma, 31, 45
malignant tumors, 136
management, 14, 25, 35, 48, 65, 75, 106, 109, 111, 114, 142, 164, 165, 166, 167
manufacturing, 101, 104
mapping, 22, 30, 46, 76, 120
mass, 15, 16, 35, 100, 105, 110, 120, 158
measles, 63, 72
measurement, 60
median, 110, 115, 117, 133, 134, 135
mediastinal, ix, x, xi, xii, 1, 3, 5, 7, 8, 14, 16, 17, 18, 19, 22, 23, 24, 25, 27, 28, 29, 30, 31, 32, 33, 35, 36, 37, 38, 39, 40, 43, 45, 46, 47, 48, 49, 51, 52, 53, 55, 56, 57, 59, 60, 62, 63, 64, 65, 66, 67, 69, 72, 75, 76, 77, 84, 85, 87, 88, 89, 91, 93, 94, 95,96, 97, 101, 102, 105, 106, 107, 109, 110, 111, 116, 119, 120, 127, 128, 133, 134, 135, 136, 137, 138, 139, 140, 141, 143, 144, 145, 146, 149, 150, 151, 152, 153, 154, 155, 157, 158, 159, 160, 161, 162, 163, 164, 165, 166, 167, 168, 169
mediastinitis, 62, 158, 162

mediastinoscopy, x, xii, 40, 149, 156, 161, 168
mediastinum, 3, 4, 5, 13, 29, 30, 31, 40, 51, 53, 102, 110, 130, 132, 135, 141, 152, 154, 155, 160, 163
medical, 20, 38, 116, 171
medicine, 133, 142, 147
medulla, 2
melanoma, 32
meningitis, 71
mesothelioma, 152, 167
meta-analysis, 79, 146
metastasectomy, 153
metastasis, 17, 18, 32, 33, 35, 45, 46, 53, 87, 120, 128, 133, 134, 135, 136, 137, 141, 154, 162, 163
metastatic cancer, xi, 33, 44
metastatic disease, 152, 154
microscopy, 69
mineralization, 36
monoclonal antibody, 111
mononucleosis, 77
morbidity, 40, 161, 162
morphology, 20, 44, 55, 130, 139
mortality, 14, 24, 81, 83, 99, 115, 161
mortality rate, 83, 115
MRI, 119
mucin, 20
muscles, 156
mutations, 23, 116
mycobacteria, 73

N

nebulizer, 67
neck cancer, 33
necrosis, 61, 90, 100, 130
neoplasm, 38
neovascularization, 116
Nepal, ix, 51, 171
nephritis, 84

neutrophils, 62
New England, 91
nodal involvement, 32, 54
nodes, 2, 4, 5, 7, 8, 10, 13, 16, 17, 18, 19, 22, 27, 29, 30, 32, 35, 36, 38, 40, 45, 54, 60, 85, 87, 89, 93, 97, 103, 110, 120, 121, 124, 126, 128, 129, 130, 131, 133, 134, 135, 136, 137, 150, 151, 152, 154, 155, 157, 158, 159
nodules, 35, 37, 63, 65, 69, 85, 86, 87, 100, 102, 103, 105
non-classical, 52
nucleic acid, 67

O

obstruction, 35
occupational lung disease, 108
opacification, 63
opacity, 103
open lung biopsy, 114
organ, 88, 90, 139, 141
organism, 61, 62, 67, 68
organs, 51
outpatient, 41, 156
ovarian cancer, 44
overlap, 139

P

pain, 14, 65, 104, 113
palliative, 23, 38
paraneoplastic syndrome, 14, 111
parenchyma, 34, 91, 94, 95, 100, 115
pathogenesis, 113, 116, 118
pathogens, 70
pathology, 2, 20, 87, 90, 163
pathophysiology, 95
pathway, xii, 13, 24
pathways, 2, 16
PCA, 48

PCR, 71, 72, 79, 113, 114, 139, 147
pemphigus, 110
penicillin, 88
perforation, 162
perfusion, 103
pericardium, 29
permission, iv, 6, 9, 17, 31, 123
pernio, 83
PET, xii, 18, 34, 37, 38, 45, 54, 57, 88, 91, 110, 112, 119, 133, 134, 135, 137, 145, 146, 150, 152, 154, 155, 163
PET CTs, xii
PET scan, 34, 37, 38, 45, 54, 57, 88, 119, 133, 154, 155
phenotype, 52
Philadelphia, 59
physicians, 22, 133, 149, 164
pigmentation, 100
plasma cells, 2, 112, 116
platysma, 156
pleura, 5, 103, 162
pleural cavity, 162
pleural effusion, 68, 116
pneumoconiosis, 36, 104
pneumonia, 66, 75, 77, 94
pneumonitis, 87, 137
pneumothorax, 41, 162
polymerase, 71, 113
polymerase chain reaction, 71, 113
population, 76, 90, 144, 147
positron, 37, 163, 164
positron emission tomography, 37, 163, 164
post-transplant, 90
prednisone, 114
pregnancy, 74
prevention, 73, 74, 78
primary biliary cirrhosis, 89
primary tumor, 16, 18, 152, 159
probe, 42, 128, 129
professionals, 48
prognosis, 20, 24, 28, 45, 52, 83, 85, 113, 115, 117, 133

project, 24, 140, 168
proliferation, 2, 101, 105, 113, 114, 116
proteins, 2
PSA, 35, 44
pulmonary alveolar proteinosis, 103
pulmonary arteries, 8
pulmonary artery, 7, 9, 42, 126, 127, 159
pulmonary function test, 85
pulmonologist, 135

response, 66, 70, 71, 82, 95, 101, 102, 113, 117, 159
rights, iv
risk, 14, 35, 36, 66, 68, 75, 81, 87, 99, 110, 116, 117, 134, 162
risk factors, 68, 75
risks, 162
rituximab, 117
RNA, 114

R

race, 83
radiation, 20, 22, 24, 38, 40, 94, 112, 153, 160
radiation therapy, 22, 24, 40
radio, 76
radiography, 14
radiotherapy, 22, 115, 167
rash, 115
reactions, 98
reactivity, 44, 70
real time, 71, 130
receptor, 23, 35, 112, 114
recognition, 104, 165, 172
recommendations, iv, 4, 23, 35, 37
recurrence, 28, 54
Registry, 142
relevance, 166
remission, 83, 85, 90, 117
renal calculi, 104
renal cell carcinoma, 31, 45
renal failure, 112
repair, 162
requirement, 90
resection, 22, 110, 159, 161
resistance, 79
resolution, 86, 99, 154
resources, 49, 129
respiratory failure, 112, 115

S

safety, 72, 129, 136, 150, 164, 169
salts, 104
sampling error, 158
sarcoidosis, 2, 29, 37, 38, 56, 81, 82, 83, 84, 85, 87, 88, 89, 90, 91, 94, 96, 137, 139, 146, 165
schooling, 171
scope, 129, 156
secrete, 82, 84
sensitivity, xii, 19, 38, 40, 54, 55, 69, 70, 71, 72, 89, 105, 133, 134, 135, 136, 137, 151, 154
sensitization, 104
sepsis, 115
sequencing, 116
serology, 69, 72
serum, 70, 84
shape, 36, 61, 76, 129, 130
shortness of breath, 64, 83
showing, 68, 71, 84, 105, 132, 138, 154
side effects, 97
signs, 2, 85
silica, 99, 101, 102
silica dust, 101
silicon, 101
silicosis, 88, 137, 140
skin, 64, 66, 81, 83, 90, 104, 111
solid tumors, 163
South Africa, 78

specialists, 38, 116
species, 78
splenomegaly, 83, 165
sputum, 64, 67, 72, 73, 74, 78
sputum culture, 72, 74
squamous cell, 20, 21, 43
squamous cell carcinoma, 20, 21, 43
standard deviation, 38
standardization, 161
state, 92, 104, 105, 106, 146
states, xi, xii, 75, 105, 114
sternum, 3, 5, 29, 124, 160
stimulation, 116
stimulus, 117
structure, 36, 51, 129, 130, 157
Sun, 138, 146
superior vena cava, 5, 124, 153, 167
superior vena cava obstruction, 153, 167
surgical resection, 22, 110, 159, 163, 169
surveillance, 28, 35
survival, 14, 16, 23, 90, 95, 96, 106, 112, 113, 115, 117, 133
survival rate, 90, 112
symptoms, 14, 15, 30, 64, 70, 72, 74, 83, 87, 101, 104, 110, 111
syndrome, 111

T

T cell, 2, 114, 116
T cell receptor, 116
T cells, 2, 114, 116
target, 89, 130
Task Force, 78
T-cell receptor, 113
techniques, 22, 67, 69, 72, 88, 114, 131, 132, 134, 141, 146, 150, 159, 161, 163, 168
telangiectasia, 111
testicular cancer, 32
testing, xii, 44, 66, 67, 70, 71, 105, 131

tetracyclines, 87
texture, 36, 61, 76
therapeutic approaches, 115
therapy, 22, 23, 54, 68, 73, 75, 76, 78, 90, 112, 114, 133, 144, 155, 158, 159, 160, 167
thoracic lymph nodes, 76, 93, 120
Thoracic lymph nodes, xi
thoracic lymphadenopathy, xii, 38, 59, 63
Thoracic lymphadenopathy, xi, 92, 106, 119, 146
thoracic surgeon, 27, 153, 161, 169
thoracotomy, 30, 32, 160, 162, 163
thorax, xi, 2, 40, 60, 136
thrombocytopenia, 110
thymoma, 110, 136
thyroid, 20, 36, 153, 156
tissue, 3, 19, 23, 34, 35, 40, 67, 69, 72, 90, 102, 110, 119, 120, 133, 139, 140, 150, 151, 156, 158, 161
toxicity, 73
trachea, 4, 5, 7, 29, 121, 124, 156, 159
tracheostomy, 153
training, 156, 172
transcription, 20
transformation, 105, 116, 117
transplant, 90, 96
transplantation, 112
treatment, 14, 16, 19, 20, 24, 28, 38, 45, 52, 53, 54, 58, 59, 64, 65, 67, 71, 73, 74, 75, 79, 86, 90, 97, 99, 108, 110, 111, 112, 113, 114, 118, 133, 150, 153, 155, 160, 163, 165, 167
trial, 91, 112, 142, 151, 154, 164, 165, 169
tuberculosis, 38, 45, 57, 61, 66, 76, 78, 79, 89, 94, 137, 138, 139, 147, 154
tumor, 13, 17, 18, 22, 23, 24, 33, 44, 51, 52, 110, 117, 128, 134, 141, 152, 157, 159, 163
tumors, 16, 17, 18, 29, 31, 36, 44, 56, 134, 136, 150, 152, 160
tunneling, 101

U

ultrasonography, 49, 89, 141
ultrasound, 19, 25, 27, 32, 33, 40, 42, 46, 47, 48, 49, 57, 67, 72, 91, 120, 129, 132, 141, 142, 143, 145, 146, 147, 150, 160, 165, 169
uniform, 16
United States, 62, 63, 78, 112, 143
urine, 71
USA, 171
uveitis, 83

V

vagus, 29
vagus nerve, 29
validation, 107
variables, 97
vein, 5, 7, 9, 124, 127, 157, 158
ventilation, 162
ventricular fibrillation, 162
vertebrae, 3, 29, 124

vessels, 1, 2, 8, 29, 160, 162
viruses, 75
vision, 156
visualization, 89, 130, 150, 156, 157
vitamin D, 84

W

water, 82
weight loss, 64, 65, 67, 83, 104, 111, 115
White Paper, 47
WHO, 49, 57
workers, 101
workplace, 82
World Health Organization, 25, 74
worldwide, 24, 81
wound infection, 162

Y

yeast, 70
yield, 19, 55, 57, 69, 71, 78, 114, 129, 131, 136, 138, 139, 142, 160, 164

Related Nova Publications

Advances in Medicinal Chemistry Research

Editor: Edeildo Ferreira da Silva-Júnior

Series: New Developments in Medical Research

Book Description: *Advances in Medicinal Chemistry Research* is a book addressed to undergraduate and postgraduate students, where recent advances in the discovery and development of effective agents against the most remarkable wide-reaching diseases are presented, divided into seven chapters.

Hardcover ISBN: 978-1-53616-368-1
Retail Price: $195

Mastitis: Symptoms, Triggers and Treatment

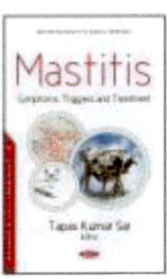

Editor: Tapas Kumar Sar

Series: New Developments in Medical Research

Book Description: The present book is a comprehensive attempt to cover the relevant topics of bovine mastitis such as physiology of milk secreation with associated biomarkers, immune responses of udder, updated etiology, current trends in conventional treatment and management, prospect of herbal preparations and propolis as supportive treatment options.

Hardcover ISBN: 978-1-53616-124-3
Retail Price: $230

To see a complete list of Nova publications, please visit our website at www.novapublishers.com

Related Nova Publications

PALLIATIVE CARE: THE ROLE AND IMPORTANCE OF RESEARCH IN PROMOTING PALLIATIVE CARE PRACTICES: REPORTS FROM DEVELOPING COUNTRIES. VOLUME 3

EDITOR: Michael Silbermann

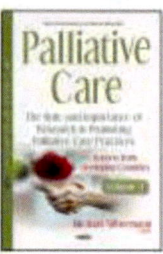

SERIES: New Developments in Medical Research

BOOK DESCRIPTION: This book owes its origins in large measure to physicians and nurses in 30 countries globally, who decided to devote their time, energy, compassion and goodwill, to the promotion of palliative care in their countries and communities, yet they lack solid evidence-based data to rely upon while extending their treatment to both patients and family members.

HARDCOVER ISBN: 978-1-53616-211-0
RETAIL PRICE: $230

PALLIATIVE CARE: THE ROLE AND IMPORTANCE OF RESEARCH IN PROMOTING PALLIATIVE CARE PRACTICES: REPORTS FROM DEVELOPED COUNTRIES. VOLUME 2

EDITOR: Michael Silbermann

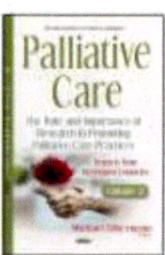

SERIES: New Developments in Medical Research

BOOK DESCRIPTION: This book owes its origins in large measure to physicians and nurses in 30 countries globally, who decided to devote their time, energy, compassion and goodwill, to the promotion of palliative care in their countries and communities, yet they lack solid evidence-based data to rely upon while extending their treatment to both patients and family members.

HARDCOVER ISBN: 978-1-53616-199-1
RETAIL PRICE: $230

To see a complete list of Nova publications, please visit our website at www.novapublishers.com